From
Bob & Ettie
Oct 17 1960

Thomas A. Dooley, M.D.

THE NIGHT THEY BURNED THE MOUNTAIN

Farrar, Straus & Cudahy · New York

Library of Congress catalog card number: 60-9079

First Printing March, 1960
Second Printing April, 1960
Third Printing May, 1960
Fourth Printing June, 1960

Published simultaneously in Canada by
Ambassador Books, Ltd., Toronto

MANUFACTURED IN THE UNITED STATES OF AMERICA
BY AMERICAN BOOK-STRATFORD PRESS, INC., NEW YORK

THE NIGHT THEY BURNED THE MOUNTAIN

Books by Dr. Dooley

DELIVER US FROM EVIL

THE EDGE OF TOMORROW

THE NIGHT THEY BURNED THE MOUNTAIN

DOCTOR TOM DOOLEY, MY STORY (*juvenile*)

To My Mother

with deep gratitude for giving me her tender love as a shield against life's winds and storms.

To Dwight Davis and Earl Rhine

with whom I've shared joys and worries, disappointments and quiet triumphs in the fog-shrouded valley of Muong Sing.

The author wishes to express his thanks to Miss Erica Anderson for the use of her photographs. All but two of the pictures in the thirty-two page insert between pages 64 and 65 were taken by her.

CONTENTS

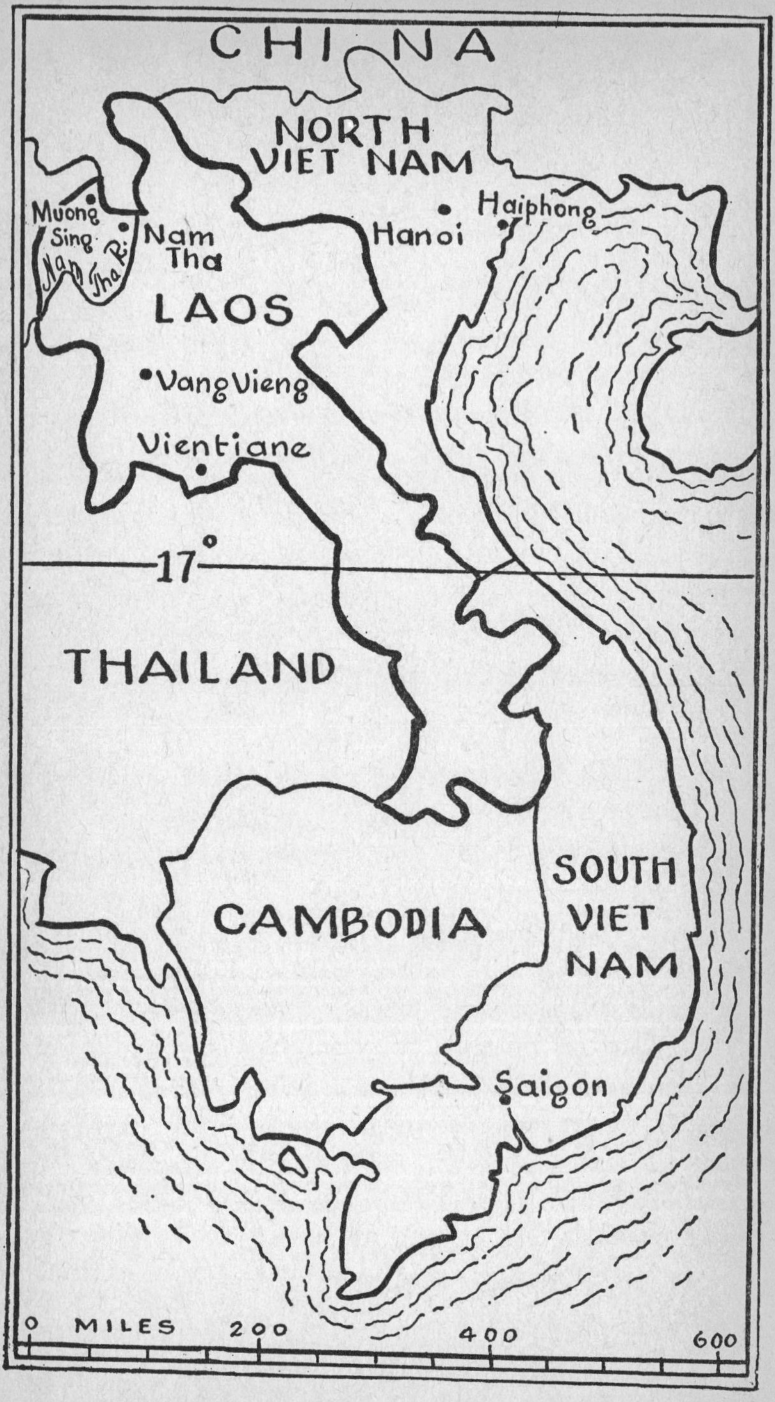

CHINA
NORTH VIET NAM
Haiphong
Hanoi
Muong Sing
Nam Tha
Nam Tha R.
LAOS
Vang Vieng
Vientiane
17°
THAILAND
CAMBODIA
SOUTH VIET NAM
Saigon
0 MILES 200 400 600

ONE ·

BEFORE MY HIGHEST MOUNTAIN

It was a Saturday, at high noon, when the tired-looking Lao soldier came into my clinic in the little village of Muong Sing in northern Laos. He snapped to a slightly languid salute and said, "*Thanh Mo America, mi tayah.* Doctor America, you have a telegram."

What could this mean? Coming on the military radio, it must be about the war. My heart jumped a little and with a dry mouth I said, "*Ou he kai.* Give it to me."

He said that it was being held at the radio shack in the fortress, and I should accompany him there. I turned the line of patients over to Earl Rhine, one of my assistants, and walked out into the rain, across the road to the fortress.

There was war in Laos, and there were rumors of more war. Only four days before, the Voice of America had broadcast that over four thousand Red troops were in the two provinces of Sam Neua and Phong Saly. Other troops were massing on the Vietnamese side of the frontier and a new attack was expected. Would it spread to the China frontier? Would we be able to go on practising medicine much longer in this little village located at a point where Laos, China, and Burma meet?

In the mud radio-shack another Lao soldier thrust a flimsy,

crumpled sheet of blue paper into my hand. He said it had been forwarded from the Lao Army headquarters in the capital. He was sorry he was so many hours late in getting it to me but "*het punh,*" the war, you know. This limp piece of paper was to become a turning-point in my life. Noon, Saturday, August 15, in the year 1959.

My knees were shaking. I sat down on the wooden bench beside the radio operator, and smoothed out the thin blue paper on the table. I tried to make out the sentences. As the Lao language has no Roman letters, French is used in telegraph messages. Each letter of the telegram was in a box by itself. When I wrote out the message with its long introductory order to the local Commandant, the part addressed to me looked like this:

FROMPE TER COMAND URAS DOCTOR DOOLEY URGENT RETURN TOUS IMMEDIATELY

The message made no sense to me. I asked that it be retransmitted. The operator said that this would take hours, but I insisted. I went back to the clinic and showed the garbled words to the boys. Dwight Davis, my other assistant, took out a pencil and immediately divided the letters so that the sentence read in English as follows:

FROM PETER COMANDURAS: DOCTOR DOOLEY, URGENT RETURN TO U. S. IMMEDIATELY

How quickly Dwight grasped and understood that telegram —how strangely quick.

Suddenly the earth seemed to open up underneath me. Return to the U. S. now? I was intending to go in three months anyway. Why *now*? Had something happened to my mother? Had something bad happened to MEDICO? Had the Ambassador to Laos notified the State Department of my refusal to leave and had they in turn requested Dr. Peter Comanduras, as chief of MEDICO, to order me out? Why didn't Peter explain himself? Why did he just say "Urgent, return to U. S.?" Didn't he know that we were involved in a war? Didn't he know that the wounded might start flowing into this hospital tomorrow? Didn't he know that the mountains of Laos were on fire? What could be so urgent that I must come home *now*, instead of when I was due to go home in a few months? Didn't Peter know that Laos was moving deeper and deeper into the shadows? This was not the time to abandon my work. Didn't he know what the Communists would say if I deserted my hospital? "A typical American reactionary imperialistic coward."

I had complete confidence in Doctor Peter Comanduras as Chief of MEDICO, but why was he ordering me out now, without explanation? He was living in the civilized world. I was living in the world beyond. More than mere miles separated us. How could he judge what must be done when he was not on the scene? It seemed to me that the sky was full of the sound of thunder. It seemed to me that the night was coming at high noon. "Urgent Doctor Dooley return to U. S. immediately." This meant that I must abandon my hospital, abandon all I had done, abandon all the work of the last year. "Urgent, return to U. S. immediately." The letters in that telegram stared up at me and stabbed my soul.

The things that I felt in my heart I said with my mouth. I asked all these questions of my two Texan assistants, Earl and Dwight. They offered no answers. They didn't even try to present anything good, except that Earl said, "Maybe you're going home to do a TV show," at which I growled back in anger.

The message had been sent by the Lao army. How did they get it? Why did Peter wire me through the Lao army?

Why didn't he send the telegram through the usual civilian channels? The army had filed it as TOP SECRET, URGENT. Had the message come so marked from America? How did it get to the Army in the first place? Was it sent to the Ambassador who requested the army to forward it to me? I was terribly concerned. My mind began to conjure up monstrous thoughts. Could it possibly have anything to do with the small tumor that Dr. Van Valin had cut off my chest? At once I banished that thought as sheer impossibility.

I decided that the wire must have something to do with the economic situation of MEDICO. It seemed to me that we were always on the brink of broke. I was going to have to go home and raise money. This infuriated me. Several times during the night I woke up suddenly, startled. I sat up in my bunk when thoughts came crowding to my mind. I did not sleep that night, nor the next night, nor for many nights to follow. By mid-week I had convinced myself that Dr. Comanduras had had a heart attack and that I was going to have to go and work at our MEDICO office. I, jungle physician, would have to sit at a desk in a New York office.

I sent a telegram down to Vientiane to Horace Smith, the American Ambassador, on Sunday. I asked him if he would please send up a plane to take me out. This was difficult to ask because only a few days before I had sent him a message pointing out that I was autonomous and that we could take care of ourselves despite the threat of war in our village. Now I had to reverse myself and ask him for his plane. I was sure the Ambassador knew about the New York telegram because I decided in my confused mind that the Lao government had received it from him.

No plane came Sunday, no plane came Monday, no plane came Tuesday. I felt as though I was tightly sealed in a coffin, my valley gray and grim. I walked around my village and talked to the people to explain to them that I had to leave quickly. They could not understand. They asked if I was afraid of the war. I tried to explain to them why I must go home, though I did not know myself. How could I explain to other ears what my own heart did not know?

On Tuesday afternoon the horizon could only be seen in dim outline; the mountains were veiled in the mist. No plane could come in now. Soon black clouds would roll across the heavens again and we would be surrounded by the monsoon storm of wind and water. These were wild and gloomy times, wild and gloomy in the valley, wild and gloomy in my heart. Yet this dirty, barren, underdeveloped Asian village of stink and misery and wretchedness suddenly seemed warm and good and close. I did not want to leave it. I did not want to abandon it. I did not want to go to America now. I could feel the dampness of soggy sentimentalism taking hold of me.

I thought, "Now, Dooley, you've got a job, and it doesn't necessarily mean that you must stay in this village. You must go where you can do the greatest good." But deeper inside me a voice said, "Stay in your village, stay wrapped in the love of being needed. Here Asians need you and you need that need." I remembered the words of a Chinese philosopher who said that life was like a tightrope. On this tightrope man walks, balanced between what he must do and what he wishes to do. If these two remain in perfect balance, he can walk forward on the rope with ease. If they do not remain in balance, he falls down on one side or the other. I must keep walking, I must walk straight forward. I must.

Suddenly, while we were sitting at a very late lunch, we heard the unmistakable drone of a small twin-engine plane. We rushed out of the house and looked up. We could see no hole in the murky clouds where the plane could pierce into our valley. I grabbed a small brief-case that I had packed and went out to the airstrip and waited. I could hear the plane as it circled and circled almost as though the fury of its engines would dispel the clouds. And they did, just as Chinese firecrackers dispel evil spirits. The Ambassador's small Beechcraft landed on our airstrip and out climbed my friend Bob Burns of USIS. There were no other passengers.

I asked Bob immediately if he knew what had happened, or why. He said, "All I know is that the Ambassador received a telegram from you saying you must leave immediately. He wishes to help and so he sent his plane. He told me to tell you that if you want to take your crew out, there is plenty of room on the plane. If you wish to leave your crew here, you must remember the immense responsibility that you place on them." "Who said that specifically?" I asked. He repeated, "The Ambassador himself." I was faced with another decision which I could not make alone. More fear.

I turned to Dwight and Earl and said, "Then this is your decision too, boys. You can get on this plane and leave with me, stay in the capital until we find out what this is all about, or you can stay here and continue to work alone." Without any hesitation they said, "Doctor, you go on, we will stay here and take care of things until you come back." I thanked God for men like mine. Yet involuntarily a hideous picture flashed in my mind—the impaled heads along the village airstrip which a French pilot had told me about. What if Earl and Dwight were captured by the Communists and beheaded as imperialistic Americans?

Dwight interrupted this ghastly thought by saying, "Do you want to take this, sir?" He held out a large crucifix given to me when I was made an honorary Oblate of Mary Immaculate. The Pope himself had blessed it and handed it to me. I said, "Why should I take it with me now? You keep it here in my house where it belongs. I will be back real soon." Dwight was again being solicitous, kind and good—something which I did not at the time understand. Instead I was depressed, angry, and irritable.

The plane revved up its motors. As it took off, I looked back at two young men standing on the very rim of Red hell, under the threat of war. Surrounding them were my nurses and interpreters who had come out to the airfield to say goodbye to me, each with more sadness in his voice than I ever remembered at a normal departure. I did not understand this. At that time I did not know what it meant.

The plane slowly corkscrewed its way up to gain enough altitude to jump the rim of the mountain. I watched the boys below until the mist swirled around and I could no longer see them. In their hearts was the same great spirit that made people cross the plains of America years ago. It is the same spirit that can keep this world free for free men to live in.

The plane flew high towards the capital. I spoke to Bob Burns. In quick words I poured out my fear, my anguish, my concern. Why, why, why? Bob kept putting his hands on my shoulders and saying, "Now don't worry about it, doctor. Don't give it another thought; you are probably going to be on a TV show." I said, "If Peter ordered me out of Laos just to appear on some TV show, I would use adjectives on the network that would shut TV down forever. I mean it."

Bob just smiled, and tried to change the subject, without success. I kept vocalizing the fear in my heart, and took refuge in wordy violence.

The plane landed at Vientiane's military airport and a car was waiting to take me to the house of absent Hank Miller. There I changed my clothes. Hank was in Bangkok, his house was full of war correspondents, and I had no desire to talk to anybody. Bob Burns told me the Ambassador had invited me to dinner so I cleaned up, put on my only suit, slightly mildewed, and walked to the Ambassador's house.

To my surprise I found that just the Ambassador, the Deputy Chief of Mission and I were to have dinner. I discussed all my fears again. Each listened to me with the patience of a father. I did not know at that time that the Ambassador was fully aware of why I was going home to America. Bob Burns knew, Hank Miller knew, Earl, Dwight and all of my crew knew. The point was, Tom Dooley did not!

I told the Ambassador that I wanted to get to Bangkok as soon as possible in order to telephone to the United States and find out what this was all about. I said, "Maybe I won't have to go home. Maybe I can handle this whole thing over long-distance telephone for a couple of hundred dollars instead of spending fifteen hundred dollars for an around-the-world plane ticket."

The Ambassador said kindly, "Tom, go ahead home for a few weeks. If you fly jets you can go home, do what you have to do, and return quickly."

The next plane to Bangkok was at five the following evening and the Ambassador said, "My plane can take you down in the morning, it is going to be going down early, and we will be glad to make room for you." I thanked him and went back to Hank Miller's for the night. I did not sleep at all. At dawn I got up and walked along the edge of the river.

In the mist of early morning I went to Mass in the Catholic church of Vientiane. Once again I heard the same familiar words in Latin, "*Ad Deum qui laetificat.* To the altar of God I will go, to God who is the joy of my youth." These are the same words I have heard in the cathedrals of Paris, of

St. Louis, of Rome, and in the village chapels of Laos and Viet Nam. These same words in Latin had given me peace and solace when I was plunged into the hideousness and atrocity of Northern Viet Nam in 1954. These words had given me comfort in the strain and stress of medical school. These words had given me faith as a young man. Why did they seem to give me little solace now?

At eight o'clock the next morning I was at the airport once again, good Bob Burns acting as driver and friend. He put me on the Ambassador's plane and by nine-thirty we were winging our way across the emerald green paddies of the Korat plains of Thailand. Two hours later we landed at the sleek international airport at Bangkok. Some friends from the Thai airlines office met me and drove me to a hotel in town. I went immediately to the post-office building to place a phone call to America. I spent most of the afternoon trying to get a call through. I had to get through, I had to find out —four days of not knowing was already taking its toll. I had neither eaten a square meal nor held down much liquid; the agony of not knowing was the most terrible thing I had ever undergone.

My chest was sore from Dr. Van Valin's surgery. The fact that my whole shoulder ached must, I thought, have been due to the long flights.

By seven that evening it was obvious that I would not be able to get my phone call through, so I telephoned the airport and told them that it was urgent that I get to Hong Kong immediately. Although Hong Kong was not in the direct route to New York, it was only a six-hour flight and telephone connections out of Hong Kong are always good.

They said they could put me on a midnight plane. I took a taxi to the hotel where I put on the only white shirt I had brought with me, and then went to a small restaurant that I liked in Bangkok.

After a miserable dinner there (it kept bouncing in my stomach) I asked the owner if I could play the piano. I frequently spent time there whenever I was in Bangkok and always played their piano. I tried to dissipate the tensions that were in me through the dexterity of my fingers and through the warmth of Chopin. However, Chopin did not seem to help, nor did Schumann, nor did anything which was soft and light and airy. I soon found myself playing the crashing chords of Rachmaninoff and the thundering opening of Tchaikowsky's concerto. After two hours of playing, some people who were sitting at a shadowy table in the corner came over within the circle of the light and said: "Hi, Tom, how are you?"

I looked up and saw the faces of my close friends, Hank Miller, and his wonderful wife, Annie. Never was I so glad to see friends as at that moment. I said I wanted to talk to them right away, I was so worried, so concerned. They said, "Don't worry, Tom; play something soft and light and lilting." I tried, but I could not make my fingers play like this. I hurt in my heart, in my shoulder, in my side. I was tired, I was sick, I was worried.

We went back to Hank's table and Hank looked at me and said, "Tom, I have never seen you in this state, even during wars, even during crisis. What's wrong?" I let flood out of my head and heart the things that had come to pass, the fear which existed because I did not know.

Hank looked at me and coolly said, "I know why you are going home. I will tell you, Tom." I leaned forward, took a deep breath and pleaded, "What's wrong, Hank?" My tension was at its peak. I thought I would burst. Slowly, deliberately, he said, "The tumor that Dr. Van Valin removed has been diagnosed as a secondary stage of malignant melanoma."

I had no reaction. The words entered my head like a fist jammed into a pillow. I felt nothing. I neither felt elation at finding that MEDICO was not in a state of chaos, nor did I feel great dejection at finding out that I had a hideously malignant growth of cancer. It just seemed for a moment that all was quiet. All was tranquil for now. At last, I knew.

I knew? Yes, I knew, as a doctor, that malignant melanoma is one of the quickest killers of flesh and blood that is known in the history of cancer.

Looking back on that night, I do not remember much more. They drove me to the airport but I do not remember what we talked about. I only remember the warmth of Annie's goodbye embrace. I only remember the strength and warmth of Hank's handclasp and his words as I climbed the plane ramp, "We'll see you soon, Tom."

On the plane the reading lights blinked out and once again I was the sleepless traveler. By dawn the plane was in Hong Kong. Listlessly I went through Customs, took a cab and checked into a hotel. I did not want to see anybody. There was nothing that I wanted to do. No need to telephone now. I might as well get the fastest plane home.

At three p.m. on Wednesday I took a jet plane headed for London. On the plane I did a great deal of thinking. Somewhere the thought came, "Blessed are they that mourn." But there must be no black pit of melancholy, no inertness, no fog, no void. I had much to do. Now there was a new urgency.

How did this cancer come about? I had always thought the months of aching and pain in my right shoulder and chest wall were due to my fall down an embankment on my last river trip. A few weeks after the fall a small lump had grown on the side of my chest wall, but I thought it was just a cyst.

When I weighed myself on the scales at the Hong Kong airport, I found that I had lost over 30 pounds. I thought, "Is my life gutted?" I tried to think with detachment; I tried to think objectively about illness and cancer, but I am a miser of life. All I could think about was the statistic I had studied in med school, "Only about 50 percent of the people who have a malignant melanoma in the metastatic (second stage) survive a year. Less than 30 percent live two years." Yet I knew I was not going to abandon what I think is the correct thing to do in life because of shadows on a page. Nor was I going to quit this living, loving passion for life that I possess simply because of a statistic. I was not abandoning the beauty and tenderness that man can give to man, just for a statistic.

Memories surged into my mind and blocked out words, memories of my villagers and their needs. Memories of the fetid pestilence and decay of the refugee camps of Haiphong. Memories of the red humid heat of Vang Vieng. Memories of the oppressive sick call at the Nam Tha hospital.

I realized that I had become more aware of myself and my soul's adventure in the raw material of Asian life. There was still much to do. I must continue to do this work as long as God allows me time on this earth to do it. I must continue to be tender, for to be tender one must be courageous. Now before my own highest mountain I must be braver than ever, even though bravery is sometimes a sad song. No, my candle was not gutted.

Looking out of the window in the moon-shimmering night I felt a cloudy out-of-touchness with everything. I had a pleasant disembodiment from my own self. The physical tiredness of the trip from Muong Sing to Honk Kong had drained me. My mind put me somewhere else where I could look back at the body of Tom Dooley.

Once many years ago, as I sat on a small stool in the candlelit room of Dr. Albert Schweitzer on the banks of the Ogowe, in French Equatorial Africa, the great old gentleman said to me, "The significance of a man, Tom, is not in what he attains, but rather in what he longs to attain." I thought to myself, I must continue to long to attain.

The value of love is stronger than that of hate, and I was confident that many people loved me and the work I was doing. I must now draw new strength from the knowledge of their love, strength because I needed it. In my detachment everything suddenly became intent and vivid. I cried a bit and at one moment I laughed out loud. The woman sitting in the seat beside me asked if I was all right. I replied, "Yes, I'm just fine."

There were some hours on that plane trip when I was surfeited with contentment, for I felt as though I had completed a job well done. The plane roared on east, flying over Thailand, Burma, India and up through Europe.

I thought about the kind of village medicine that I was doing. It would be hard for me to do anything else. This kind of medicine is my salvation, my hold on life. It is my means of expression. Also flowing and surging in me was the passionate desire to tell others of this work, of this kind of medicine, of this life. I did not see how I could ever quit village work. I must treat patients with my own hands, reach out and give personal help every day. I feel that I must go out of my way to do it and to do it with tenderness.

I thought of Earl and Dwight back at work in Muong Sing. And I thought of my other crews in former years. And one thing stirred me, the fact that so many people gave me something or were something to me without my knowing it. There were some people I had never exchange a word with, but had merely heard of by report. There were others that I had known and loved. All these people had a decisive influence on me. They entered into my life and became a power within me, almost without my knowledge.

I had left Muong Sing so rapidly that I had forgotten to say "So long" to the boys, at least "So long" as warmly as I would had I known I would be gone for months. I began to go over in my mind all the events of the past months. I remembered the day I arrived in Laos, and the press conference announcing the start of MEDICO which was held in New York before my departure. It was February 4, 1958. What had I said to the reporters? I must try to remember . . .

TWO ·

THE START OF *MEDICO*

"Ladies and gentlemen, a few weeks ago I turned over to my publisher the manuscript of my book, *The Edge of Tomorrow*. It ended on the encouragement of Dr. Albert Schweitzer's word of hope. When we told Dr. Schweitzer of the plan we are going to announce to you today, he accepted Honorary Chairmanship and he sent us this message: 'I do not know what your destinies will ever be, but this I do know: you will always have happiness if you seek and find, how to serve.'

"Now today, on the fourth of February, 1958, I feel as though I were on the verge of the longest journey I have ever taken."

In trying to communicate to the newsmen before me, I felt I had become a little stiff. I must grope and find *me* again. It had been so long since I had had to express myself to fellow-Americans like this. I felt a strong confidence welling up within me, forming my words. This same confidence, blended with sweat, effort and hope, must form the action of MEDICO.

"On this day a new organization is being founded. It will be entitled MEDICO, which stands for Medical International Cooperation Organization. MEDICO's reason for existence is simple. We wish to take care of people who are sick, in areas where they have little or no chance of receiving medical aid.

"We are in no way a religious or political organization. We're not intending to convert anyone to Catholicism, or Protestantism, nor are we trying to make them new Republicans or old Democrats. We are not trying to replace any already existing programs in the field of health. We feel that the World Health Organization and the International Cooperation Administration of our government's foreign aid program are doing excellent jobs in preventive medicine. What we wish to do is a job in simple therapeutic medicine."

I wondered if the meaning of therapeutic was clear. "By therapeutic I mean the simple act of passing out pills. Sometimes foreign aid becomes enmeshed in an obscure tangle of programs. The simplicity of MEDICO's program is this: we actually believe that we can win the friendship of people only by getting down on the ground and working beside them, on equal terms, humans-to-humans, towards goals that they understand and seek themselves. MEDICO is a person-to-person, heart-to-heart program. There is no more personal relationship than that of a doctor and his patient. We feel that therapeutic medicine will have a double effect: it will aid those who are sick and by that simple act it will win friendship for America."

Someone in the audience raised his hand and asked, "Where did the idea of MEDICO come from?"

"The idea of MEDICO is a blend of three ideas. We have taken some of the philosophy of Dr. Schweitzer, who believes that man belongs to man, that man has claims on man, and we have given it today's accent. We feel that man has claims on man but that this idea must be modernized into a program of self-help, a program that produces something *now*—

today and tomorrow, not next year or next decade. That dream of Schweitzer's was part of my work in the small village of Nam Tha in Laos. We tried to show the villagers of Nam Tha that we five Americans really believed that Asians had claims on us. We left America to go live amongst them, to be an intimate and integral part of their community life. In Nam Tha we cared for thousands of their sick and wounded. We delivered their babies, we went to their weddings and their funerals, and we joked with their young military. We tried to show, with love, that we understood the responsibility of those who have towards those who have not.

"We therefore added a little modern touch to this fundamental philosophy, and in correspondence with Dr. Peter Comanduras we matured this idea. Dooley and his boys can care for about 36,000 people a year; however, there are about 36 million times some other multiple who still need help. We should really enlarge our program. When I returned to America just a few months ago, Dr. Peter Comanduras and I met in Washington and we talked about our mutual dreams. It was from this that MEDICO was born.

"Dr. Peter Comanduras is the Secretary General of our program. He has superb abilities that will earn for our program the position of respect it deserves among our fellow-Americans. He is giving up his private practice and teaching to devote all of his time and talent to MEDICO. He is making a great sacrifice.

"On the village level, I have had several years of practice and experience. Both of our lives are permeated with the Schweitzer concept of brotherhood. This is the combination that gave birth to MEDICO.

"In summing it up, let me say this—MEDICO wishes to render a service to people of foreign lands and at the same time render service to our own country. We wish to clear up some of the fears and misconceptions of America that are held by people of some foreign lands. We wish to take care of their sick, and in return we wish only their love and understanding. We believe that medicine is above the give-and-take of national rivalry.

"Dr. Comanduras is leaving immediately on a tour of the world. On this tour he will speak to the leading medical people of many nations to see if they can utilize the services of MEDICO.

"I'm leaving on a lecture tour in order to raise three things: men of medicine to work in the various MEDICO teams around the world. Second, the medicines and surgical supplies that our village hospitals will need. And thirdly, the dollar donations from the general public upon which MEDICO must exist."

Then the questions started . . .

"No, MEDICO will not necessarily work in Asia alone but in any nation that asks us."

"Yes, MEDICO will demand much from the host nation. They must give free Customs entry, furnish internal transportation, kerosene, gasoline, give us *carte blanche* for their medical warehouse. Most important, the host nation must promise to sustain and maintain what we establish, after our departure."

"Yes, the host government will also be asked to pay indigenous salaries."

"How long will our teams stay in one area? That depends. In Laos I believe that we can build a hospital, stock it, run this hospital, train the personnel to handle it, and turn it over to them within a period of two to four years. In other areas this length of time might be longer."

As quickly as it had started, the press conference ended.

Peter and I looked at each other, took a deep breath, and then realized what lay ahead of us—many months of begging, of organization, of talking. We had built our castle in the air. Now we must put a solid foundation under it.

I left the very next day to begin a lecture tour of America, covering all parts of the country. I spoke in high schools, in women's clubs, in medical societies. I spoke to people on trains and planes. Everywhere I tried to point out how MEDICO does not conflict with any existing organization. I stayed in cheap hotels in small towns, in magnificent suites in large cities. The lecture tour consisted of 188 speeches in 79 different cities over 5 months.

I went to the leading pharmaceutical houses of America, and once again they demonstrated their great generosity. Chas. Pfizer & Co., Mead Johnson & Co., and Eli Lilly & Co. were especially generous to me as they always had been in the past. We set up MEDICO in the beginning as a division of the International Rescue Committee. We needed a mother organization to help us get started. Through the good offices of the International Rescue Committee we acquired a warehouse, and soon the medicines and supplies began to pour in. Later we became an independent organization.

The A. S. Aloe Company of Saint Louis, Missouri, supplied me once again with all the surgical equipment that we needed. Their Vice President, Henry Scherck, became MEDICO's most powerful friend. He headed our Committee for Procurement of Surgical Supplies.

When my lecture tour was finished in June, MEDICO had over one million dollars worth of medicines donated to it, and about three hundred thousand dollars in cash donations. My book, *The Edge of Tomorrow,* was condensed in "The Reader's Digest" in the issue of May, 1958. This brought a tremendous response in dollars, and also illuminated the purpose of MEDICO to millions of people around the world. Everywhere I went in America people showed their warm admiration towards our program—warm admiration portrayed by cold cash.

Over six hundred doctors, corpsmen and nurses had applied to join the various MEDICO teams. I had started out to raise money, men and medicine. And with the luck of the Irish and the grace of God, MEDICO had these three. After the tour ended, Dooley was nearly voiceless. Well, almost. When Peter returned from his round-the-world tour, he told me we had been invited by 23 nations of the world to do our kind of work in their nations.

It had been at the end of 1957, after turning my hospital at Nam Tha over to the Lao government (the story I tell in *The Edge of Tomorrow*), that I had come home, via Africa. In Lambarene I had one of the greatest privileges of my life—working at the hospital of Dr. Albert Schweitzer. And there I had dreamed up and solidified much of the plan for a world-wide miracle: MEDICO! Now that our plan was really launched, I would soon leave for Laos once again.

THREE ·

PICKING A NEW MEDICAL TEAM

I was pleased and grateful that over six hundred men and women had written in the opening months to volunteer to work with me in Laos or on other MEDICO teams around the world. Yet how would I ever choose my new men? This would be a risky thing. My last team was made up of men with whom I had worked before. They had been my Navy corpsmen, I knew what they were like. I knew that their abilities and friendship would be a help to me. For the new team I would have to choose unknown, untried men, and this would be really difficult.

Throughout the lecture tour, after each speech, people would come up and say, "Doctor, I'd like to do that kind of work with you in Asia. I am an ex-Army or ex-Navy corpsman. May I help you?" I would always set up plans to have breakfast with them, or coffee later on. After I spoke with them, I would go back and write prodigious notes about each person, covering everything from their personalities to their medical and surgical abilities.

The choice of Earl Rhine and Dwight Davis was almost accidental. On March 17th, *Life* magazine did a picture story on my lecture tour. Two young men working in a hospital in Austin, Texas, read that story, turned and said to each other,

"This is the kind of work for us." Both these men were veterans, and both were surgical technicians working at Brackenridge Hospital while in pre-med at the University of Texas.

They then sat down and composed a lengthy letter of application, including a list of every single surgical experience that they had had, every operation on which they had assisted, and all of their sundry talents. Then they slept on it and in the morning they decided the letter was no good. They then wrote a very terse and succinct letter, offering their services to me and asking for an immediate reply.

They went one step further. They telephoned my mother. The fact that they obtained her number and had the intelligence to find the city in which she lived was a pleasing thing to me. My mother has a very good sense of business about her and endorsed the boys practically by "the sound of their voices" and their go-to-itiveness.

Their letter came to me like all the other letters, but when I saw the Texas address I telephoned Pete Kessey, one of my old crew who lived in Austin. I asked Pete to interview these two volunteers. I pointed out to Pete that he must give only the blackest picture of working in Asia, and especially point out what a hard-headed, stubborn, difficult and irascible son-of-a-gun Dooley was to work for.

The next night Pete called me and said he'd interviewed these two men and thought "they were both tops." Knowing me as well as he did and knowing what these two men would be involved in, working and living with me, Pete was an excellent judge. After all, like most humble Irishmen, I think I'm practically faultless. Pete does not exactly agree, so he could warn potential candidates about the guy for whom they would work. I didn't want some juvenile enthusiast who would sour and quit on me when proximity dulled the edge of admiration.

A week later I called the men and set up an appointment in Houston, Texas. I had a speech in New York on a Monday and in Washington on a Wednesday, so that gave me all of Tuesday free. I took an early morning plane on Tuesday and arrived in Houston, where Earl and Dwight met me at the airport.

They told me many months later, with a laugh in their voices, how they stood so nervously at the ramp, watching various people get off the plane. Earl would say, "That's him," and Dwight would respond, "Oh, no, he's too fat." Then Dwight would say, "Maybe that's him," and Earl would reply, "Oh, no, he's too old." Their nervousness led in this guessing game. Finally they did spot me and I spotted them. My first impression was, "These guys are too well dressed to work for me in a dirty Asian village."

Yet after about four hours of speaking with them, I had made up my mind that these were the men I wanted. They were the best of any I had interviewed. They possessed innumerable qualities that I wanted. They were not in any way religious fanatics and their idealism was balanced by a sense of realism because, in their overseas' duties they had seen the stink and misery in which idealism must rub its nose. Yet they had enough youthful idealism to be willing to accept the challenge of any kind of a job. They were in good health and had superb medical technician training.

They both were seniors at the University of Texas and wanted to go on to become doctors. They had an obvious amount of admiration for Tom Dooley, yet neither was too full of hero worship. They seemed, after a four-hour interview, to have a good sense of balance between right and wrong, duty and pleasure. My own opinion, blended with what Pete had told me and my mother's intuitive knowledge, convinced me that these were my new crew. We then went to dinner at a glorious hotel in Houston to enjoy the first meal that we would ever have together, including the last steak that we would eat together for a long time.

Several times during the conversation I mentioned that they both had on the same kind of dark blue pin-stripe necktie. Each time I mentioned it, they gulped. Later, Dwight asked, "Doctor, would it make any difference if we were married?" I said, "Of course it would. I would not take a married man with me. On my last trip, Denny Shepard and Norm Baker were married. Things were doubly tough for them than for the bachelors of my team. I feel that to do this kind of work one must devote to it all his time, all his energy, and all his emotions. He could not be involved with nostalgia and homesickness for wife and family."

Dwight again said, "You mean that if we were married you would not take us?" To which I replied, "Probably not. Why? You're certainly not married, are you?"

With this they both slumped in their chairs, took a deep breath, and said, "Yes, we are both married."

They proceeded to spend the next hour, explaining how happy their wives were that they were going to Asia. This I found hard to believe. They insisted. They said they had no children and both their wives were working independently and would continue their nursing work. Their wives said that their salaries and the $150 a month I planned to pay the boys would be enough. Earl was quick to point out that he'd been married seven years though only 26, and "we are not exactly honeymooners, sir." I had been convinced that these were the top men of all that I had interviewed. I was pleased with Pete's opinion of them, so once again I decided that I'd better change my mind. After all, isn't changing one's mind a sign of intelligence?

At dinner I again commented that they looked like the Bobbsey Twins with their identical neckties. They burst out laughing and said, "We wore these neckties at Dwight's wedding several years ago. By accident we both put them on tonight, and almost let the cat out of the bag when you noticed that they are identical."

We smiled that evening and laughed with the warm laughter that comes from good companionship. I took a midnight plane back to the east and the boys drove back to their homes in Austin. The decision was made. Their wives were not opposed to their doing this kind of work as they intelligently realized what fine men this experience would make them. My team was formed. All of us were happier men by dawn that next day.

Dwight Davis is 27 years old. He was born and raised in the state of Washington. While he was in the Air Force, he was stationed in Korea. He had plenty of time to see some of the wretchedness into which he was now plunging his life, the wretchedness of Asia. In 1955, as a civilian, he started college in Austin, Texas, and began to work nights at Brackenridge Hospital. It was at that time that he met a fellow veteran, Earl Rhine. Dwight and Earl became fast friends and this friendship was one of the things that pleased me about their application. "They sound like a good pair. Two for the price of one," I thought to myself. I smiled because I thought it was good to have a pair. It is good for two men who work together to be friends because they would have mutual solace when I got angry with one, and angry I do get.

Dwight is tall and very slender, with a tightness in his facial features. When his horn-rimmed glasses slip down off his nose a bit, he looks something like Arthur Miller. With an immobile face he sometimes seems stern, but he is not at all; quite the contrary. He has a heart so big that it suffuses his character. He has a wonderful love for children. He calls village kids "Mr. Bigger-eyes-than-mine" or "Tex" or "Hi, buddy." Dwight walks with a lithe gait, but in a long and lanky step, not unlike a Texan even though Texas is his adopted state. He speaks with a clipped accent of the northwest, but has adopted the expansiveness of Texans. His eyes are deep-set, penetrating, and blue in color. You rarely see them, however, because the rim of his low-slung glasses hides his eyes. His hair is close-cropped, almost a crew cut, though it gets a little long and scraggly at the back of his neck. His wife is a Mexican girl and, as a consequence, Dwight speaks good Spanish. In the mountains of Indo-China, when upset, he would break out into a spate of Spanish.

Dwight is a quiet man, and I used to think that he was almost invisible, saying very little, though always working much. In seventeen months of working with me, he never expressed any particular emotional response to having Dooley for his boss nor to working amongst these people of Asia. However, like the proverb of the way still water runs deep, I always knew that Dwight Davis was deep. Over a year later, in a hospital bed in New York, I was to receive a letter from him which proved this adage.

Earl Rhine is 26 years old. "Rhine like the river," he would say. Though born in Illinois, Earl had lived in Texas long enough to become "Texan." (In spite of this language barrier I was able to communicate with him.) After many years of marriage, just a few weeks before Earl left for Laos, he found out that his wife was pregnant. He nevertheless felt as though he could afford a year and a half out of his life to invest in Asia. He had a valiant little gal for a wife who said that she would take care of herself and their child while Earl was out taking care of thousands of kids in Asia. Indeed, she did.

Earl is shorter than Dwight. The thing about Earl that you noticed immediately was the extreme gentleness of his manner. This later became doubly obvious when I watched how he handled his patients. His black curly hair had earned him the nickname "Marcel"; he likes neither the nickname nor the hair. His features are round and though not fat he is somewhere between chubby and normal. He has large brown eyes and at six o'clock at night he looks like he should shave again. As I was later to observe with satisfaction, he does his tasks quietly and he does them well.

In Earl and Dwight I was confident I had as good a medical team as I could possibly have found to work with me in the unknown months ahead. I could soon fly towards the edge of tomorrow once more.

FOUR ·

ARRIVAL IN LAOS

In June I boarded a plane for Hawaii. MEDICO was not yet five months old. My mind was flooded with plans and my heart was warmed by the generosity of my country. I was pleased at having had contact with the abrasive minds of some of the young students of America; I was still dizzy from the questions asked by thousands of them on my lecture tour. I looked out of the window of the magnificent Pan American plane and watched a little sunlight come over America. That same sunlight would soon be over Asia. I hoped that this sunlight would warm the hearts of the people of Asia whom I had grown so to love.

As the plane swooped into the airport at Hawaii, I remembered landing here as a young Navy officer. In 1954 I first came here as a Navy doctor, just having finished my internship. I was en route to duty in Yokusuka, Japan. After only a few weeks in Japan I was transferred into the chaos that was to become the evacuation of North Viet Nam. For one year I stayed in North Viet Nam, working in a huge refugee camp. In my first book, *Deliver Us From Evil,* I told how more than 600,000 miserable, wretched and beaten but valiant people passed through my camp. I had the good fortune of being an intimate part of one of the greatest tributes to the majesty of the human spirit. I saw it, I was there. I had the joy of seeing white-capped sailors respond to a call, a need, a cry for help: North Viet Nam in 1954 and 1955!

I stayed in Hawaii a week. More Americans came to the help of MEDICO. Especially grand to me was a small group of young men and women called the Junior Chinese Catholic Club and their leader, Fred Luning. Later we were to have an even more eloquent testimonial of their effectiveness.

The following weekend Earl Rhine and Dwight Davis flew to Hawaii and spent two days. This was only the second time that I had seen them in my life. I looked at these two men and thought to myself, "Dooley, you're going to live with these two guys for two years. You had better get accustomed to them, and they to you."

In the first week of July we flew to Japan and on to Hong Kong. At the latter place we had a lot of things to buy. We spent many hours walking up and down the streets of Hong Kong, arguing over prices. The Wilson Club of Bridgeport, Connecticut, had sent me a generous donation. They had written and said that they did not want to contribute any money to MEDICO itself but rather wanted to contribute something personally to me. They asked what I would like to have. I blithely answered, "A piano so I can take Chopin to North Laos." Two months later, they sent me the money. And now in Hong Kong I must find a piano.

It was an enjoyable hunt. After several days of testing every for-sale piano in Hong Kong, I finally found the zinc-lined one I wanted. But the price was almost twice as much as the Wilson Club had sent. Fortunately, the Chinese man knew of my work (after I not-so-humbly told him about it), so he generously cut the price in half. This blessed piano proved to be my most constant friend.

We flew to Saigon, where we stayed at the orphanage of Madame Vu Thi Ngai, the gallant woman of North Viet Nam whose 500 refugee children had come with her. She was now established in her new orphanage buildings in Saigon, supported by the fine American community there. Earl, Dwight and I climbed into a newly arrived jeep, painted Kelly green, which was a gift from the Willys Corporation, and began our drive across the belly of southeast Asia.

Several days later, in Cambodia, we talked to the health officials and the American Ambassador in order to make the final preparations for our MEDICO team in Cambodia. Then we went to the ancient jungle ruin of Ankor Wat.

The first night of our arrival we went out to the pool behind the Court of the Leper King. I had loved this place from years back, and wanted to go now and take a swim under the night sky. We did, and then sat around and talked. Things seemed so tranquil here. What would the next year show? Would our new hospital in Laos be successful or would it merely be a wasted effort? Would the Communist threat become more powerful and the atrocities of Yunan, China, reach out into northern Laos? Was my former hospital at Nam Tha, which we had turned over to the government of Laos, continuing or had it already collapsed?

Were those who criticized me in southeast Asia as powerful and vitriolic in their anti-Dooley ideas as they had been in the past? Would those who could think only in terms of multi-million-dollar projects snigger at my paltry efforts, or would they see that if the darkness is black enough a small candle can give a brilliant light? But worst of all, would the ogre of Communism conquer and consume the country into which we were going to move? Sitting on the mossy stones around the side of the pool behind the Court of the Leper King, I thought of how I had grown to love these people of southeast Asia. I tried to tell Earl and Dwight of how quickly they would lose their hearts to these primitive people. I tried to tell them something of the problems that would soon face them, and I wanted to steel them for the stink and death of their next two years. We sat and talked about a realization that we all possessed—the realization that the only way man can achieve his own happiness is to strive for the happiness of others. This is a simple guide: every man has a responsibility to every other man. These two boys volunteered to go to the high rain-forest of northern Laos to act out their responsibility to other men.

I warned them of the difficulties they would encounter, hostilities from the enemy as well as green-eyed hostility from fellow Americans. I warned them of the stupidity and the ignorance, the stubbornness and the cling-to-the-pastness of the mountain tribes of northern Laos. I tried to tell them that there would be many moments in each of their days that would involve someone's very life; therefore, those moments involve eternities.

We talked of the valley of Muong Sing where we expected to work, a valley just over the mountain from Nam Tha, my former village. I told them that what comes to the valley of Muong Sing in the tide of time will affect other valleys and other lands and other people.

Earl said, "It seems so hard to realize that we are soon to be thrown into such chaos. Here at Ankor things are so tranquil."

"That is exactly the point of Asia," I said. "Earl, you will spend your days being amazed at contradictions like this. The magnificence of a wild and wonderful jungle contrasted with the wretchedness of the people who live in it; the glories of God's nature and the seeming injustices that God puts on this earth; the tranquility of a pool at the Court of the Leper King and the hideous atrocities of northern Viet Nam; the red-hot heat of a humid day and the blue cool breeze of the mountain night."

While we were swimming, Dwight noticed a gold medal around my neck and asked to see it. He read on the back of the St. Christopher medal the words that have guided my life since 1954, the words of Robert Frost:

> *"The woods are lovely, dark and deep,*
> *But I have promises to keep,*
> *And miles to go before I sleep."*

Quietly we got back into our jeep and returned to the hotel.

Two days later we arrived in Bangkok. The boys took the jeep in for its first checkup while I flew on to Vientiane, the capital of Laos. I have a warm feeling towards many of the officials and the people of Laos. And I know that they possess the same toward me. My book on their country had been successful in America, and the Lao government had formally thanked me for telling Americans something of their Kingdom, its trials, and its needs. The Lao government, both officially and as my friends, was looking forward to welcoming me back to their Kingdom. And deep in my heart I was looking forward to my return, first to the capital, and then to my old village. Although I had been gone only eight months, I felt no less near to them than I ever had. My heart was bursting as the plane landed at the hot metal landing strip at the capital. I had returned to Laos. I promised I would. Excitement made my mouth dry while sweat rolled down my body. I was the first to push out the door and down the steps.

There were no Lao to meet me. Nor were there any Americans. Was the plane early? No. Why had none of my Lao friends come to welcome me back? The chief of the United States Information Service, Hank Miller and his wife, probably my closest friends in all Asia, were on home-leave in America. I had wired my date of arrival well in advance to the USIS in Vientiane. I was checking my bags off the plane when an official American car pulled up with one of the USIS men. This official said to me, "Good heavens! Your plane came in on time. Planes never come in on time. We usually don't come out until much later." I immediately flushed with anger at this haughty attitude of the white man toward the Asians and their efforts at running an airline. I asked him, "Did you notify the Lao government of the time of my arrival?" He replied, "Oh, I intended to, but I'm awfully sorry, I never had a chance. I told one of my Lao assistants to go tell the Prime Minister, however. I don't know whether he did or not."

The next morning I went to the office of this same American and asked if he had made the requested appointment for me with the Premier. He apologized for "not having had a chance to get around to it but he would send an assistant over immediately." I said, "Don't bother." I then walked two blocks to the office of the Prime Minister and asked his secretary if I could see him. His secretary beamed excitement, and within five minutes I was sitting near my good friend, Premier Phoui Sananikone. He expressed regret that no one had met me at the airlines. He knew I was en route back to my "second home" and said, "We are very unhappy that we did not have a chance to extend to you the warm welcome and the affection that all of us hold for you, our *Thanh Mo America.*" How good to hear my old title again, "Doctor America."

I told the Premier of our new plans for the village of

Muong Sing and the new hospital there. This choice had been made by many members of his Cabinet months before my return. He told me that things in my old hospital at Nam Tha were going well. I intended to return to Bangkok the next day and drive our jeep across Thailand, straight north to the Mekong River. We would then cross on the ferry and come into Vientiane. He again said, "My King has ordered us to extend to your mission all of the facilities of his government. This we do with great pleasure." They had done exactly this for me for the previous two years.

Again they were affirming their desire to help me to help them. They pledged to me Customs-free entry, all free kerosene and gasoline, and all indigenous salaries to be paid by them. We could have medicines that they had available at their pharmacy, and any other help that I could possibly need. The Prime Minister said, "We have the enthusiasm, we have the basic potential. You bring to us your American talents and your American medicines and teach us so that we can care for our own people."

I went to spend the night at Hank Miller's home, in his absence, and there met another man who was soon to become one of my closest friends. His name was Bob Burns. He worked for USIS, though when you asked him what he did, he would modestly reply, "I'm simply a typist in the army of the Lord." As he was non-Catholic, I always kidded him that he had "the right Lord but wrong army." It was a standing joke from that day for us to call Bob Burns "simply that typist."

I visited the Minister of Health who informed me that the warehouse would be ready for us the following week so I could transship the thirty-two tons of medicines from Bangkok. In the morning I flew back to Bangkok.

The crew loaded up the jeep, arranged for the transshipment, and a few days later we drove on to Vientiane. We arrived at the river late at night, left our jeep on the Thailand side of the Mekong River and crossed over in a small boat. The outboard motor pooped out and we were swept down river in the rapid current, away from the capital of Vientiane. I smiled and thought to myself, "A fine way to introduce my two men to their new Kingdom, down the river, motorless."

However, in about fifteen minutes the motor sputtered to life again, being resuscitated by the Lao mechanic who repaired it with string, spit, sweat, and ingenuity. On the Lao side of the Mekong we hitched a ride to Hank Miller's house where Bob Burns was waiting for us with bourbon on the rocks. After a clean shower, we collapsed into bed—the first night that Earl and Dwight were to spend in Laos. They would see many, many more nights before their task was done.

By previous plans, all our equipment arrived the next day. It was brought across the river and driven on trucks up to the capital. The Lao government warehouse, where the equipment would be stored, was near the Customs House. However, things were "not quite ready" and we could not put the medicine in the warehouse. I asked the American Economic Mission if they had a warehouse available for a few days. They "regretted." I looked around town for a high enough space to store this medicine for a short length of time, but no luck. As I could not leave the medicine on the trucks, there was only one alternative. The rest of the afternoon was spent unloading thirty-two tons of equipment on the lawn around Hank Miller's house. When Bob Burns returned from work, he found Hank's house practically engulfed by thirty-two tons of crates whose cubic measurements were about the size of a solid football field, ten feet high.

While the boys were unloading (as the Commanding Officer I try to do as little physical labor as possible), I had gone to find Chai. Those of you who have read my other books know that Chai is my very good friend, corpsman, interpreter, and entrepreneur. I found Chai out near his old home on the outskirts of Vientiane. This was only a few blocks from where I had met him at a love-court, when he was courting a young girl in June, 1956. Here, two years later, Chai was now living, married to that girl.

I told Chai of our problem and he said, "*Ban pinh yanh,*" which means rustically: "To hell with it," or just about anything else you want it to mean. He immediately rounded up a half dozen of his friends and they all drove with me to Hank's house and gleefully perched themselves on top of the boxes to stand guard for the night. With no more concern than that, with complete confidence in their honesty, Earl, Dwight and I dragged ourselves into bed, the day's work done. With nearly a quarter of a million dollars worth of medicines and equipment piled around the house, covered wtih palm leaves, and guarded by Chai's languid friends, we slept well.

FIVE ·

THE VILLAGE OF MUONG SING

Muong Sing is the valley just west and a little north of Nam Tha. It is a full day's walk, but only a fifteen-minute flight, from the site of my former hospital, because the mountain which divides Nam Tha from Muong Sing rises to about 8,000 feet. Muong Sing is located just five or six miles south of the China border. It is on a direct line north from Bangkok through Vientiane to the China frontier. This is the northwest corner of northern Laos.

The almost enchanted village of Muong Sing sleeps on the floor of the valley at about 2,000 feet. All around it are purple, jagged mountains. Some of the peaks run 10,000 feet high but the average is 8,000 feet. They encircle three sides of Muong Sing, leaving only the south end of the valley open. From peak to peak is a distance of only some 25 miles.

The Prime Minister had given me a letter to the Commandant of the Lao Army, authorizing all internal transportation. That afternoon I met with the Commandant in Vientiane and chose the following morning for my reconnaissance flight to Muong Sing while the boys worked at the warehouse.

The flight from the capital to the north is a spectacular thing. Flying over the Kingdom of Laos you see craggy mountain peaks whose spires stick up into the blue sky. In the space between these spires are broad valleys, checkerboard flat. Most are filled with small, green rice paddies. Each paddy looks like a square of beads all strung together, or a tangle of beads, or beads in a row, or in a coil, or beads twisting upon each other like a rosary dropped on a flat surface. The beads of green are in dovetailing knots, and sometimes the large beads seem to engulf the small. Between each square of rice field is a small brown-black dam of earth.

In almost every valley's central portion is a small clear river. From high in the sky it looks like a small vein or artery of clear, cool water. As you look you think, "What a lovely Shangri-La," but it is not that at all. It is another unsanitary, underdeveloped Asian village.

The further north, the more mountainous the countryside becomes, and down deep in the foliage of those mountains is wild and wonderful jungle. When the plane flies low, it seems as though the trees are reaching up to grab the plane. In some areas the mountain has been burned; I was to learn a great deal about this native custom.

It is understandable why the plane must corkscrew down in order to land on the floor of the valley. Although I had spent much time flying in Asia, when the plane suddenly lurched to the starboard and began to drop into the valley, I felt my heart go up to my mouth.

The road of the Muong Sing valley is cut out of the thick green of the jungle floor. From my plane it looked like a gray bony streak. Dotted along on both sides of the road are small little clusters of huts—these are the villages. Each village has its complement of dogs, chickens, cats, and children all of whom mix together and stray around under the houses. Asian houses are built up on stilts to protect them against the mud of the rains. Also the family animals can get under the house for warmth and their odor is considered to be a sign of wealth. These villages sure are wealthy!

The village of Muong Sing at first glance is a sleepy little place. It is a typical Asian village, wretchedly underdeveloped, but rich with potential for future progress. The nearby rice paddies are flooded much of the year, and the emerald green of ripened rice is a beautiful thing.

The plane finally landed. From the airstrip one must walk about twenty minutes to get to "downtown" Muong Sing. There are really several villages for the quadrangle of Muong Sing has a village dangling on the top of each of its four corners. Muong Sing, with appendages, has about 4,000 inhabitants. Along one edge of the village is a large "Beau-Geste"-type mud fortress, complete with moat. Adjacent to the military encampment is a house of the village Mayor, or Chao Muong.

First of all, I went to see the Chao Muong. He was a nice little man, socially charming, and not very effective. He took me over to two forlorn and dilapidated straw-mud-cement huts. "Our dispensary," he said. So these were the buildings that would be turned over to us to rebuild and to make into a hospital! This was not a new challenge. It was just as it had been in Nam Tha not so long ago. I had only to look at the buildings to know how much work stood ahead. I checked on the nearness of the water supply (it was far away), and the nearness of the military (very close). In fact, our hospital would be across the road from the fortress. I wondered how much aid the languid-looking Chao Muong would give to us.

A few hours later I flew out of the valley. The plane plunged into the misty evening sky, just skimming the treetops. It then circled over up and up and finally leveled out and rode on the very crest of the jungle for just a moment. It suddenly banked tightly, making one more circle in order to rise above the crest, and vaulted over the mountains on to the south. I looked at the horizon ahead and it seemed to sink and slowly rotate, and suddenly we were in the marshmallow mist of the clouds. I looked again at the valley below, jeweled and precise. It lay quietly. It seemed tranquil. Would it be this way for long, I wondered, or would war soon wound it and burn it and scar it? In less than three hours the plane took me back to the heat of Vientiane.

In the capital we then went to work, loading planes to bring equipment to the north. I knew it would take about eight round trips and so we planned to take the first load of essential living equipment up and leave Earl, Dwight, Chai and Si, my former chief cook and bottle washer, who had rejoined us. I would return on the empty plane. The following day I could return to the north with another load, and back again. By this process we figured that within a week we could move about eight tons of essential equipment and medicines to start our project. The remaining 24 tons would be brought up as needed, over the ensuing months.

The next morning at dawn we loaded two tons onto borrowed trucks and drove to the military airport just outside the city of Vientiane. We loaded the planes. Earl and Dwight spent much of their time on this flight north looking out of the windows. They were heading to the village where they had come to invest two years of their lives. As the plane flew northward, their tension built and mine did too. Several hours later we bounced to a landing on the thick grass strip of Muong Sing.

We then unloaded the plane, but we were not alone. We had the help of many villagers who were all watching and wondering what this spectacular thing that had come to them really was. They would soon know. From the landing strip into town there is a trail. On either side of the trail there is a high wall of jungle trees, almost inextricable vegetation. There is always a soft and sweetish smell in this valley, and almost always strange and savage sounds. While the villagers were unloading the plane, under the direction of Chai and Si, Dwight, Earl and I walked fast into town. I wanted to show them the huts that would be ours.

Earl and Dwight were aghast. The main house in which we were to live had just a yawning hole instead of a door. The floor was sunken and there were pools of brackish water in the center of each room. There was a cesspool-like area that I wanted converted into the kitchen. On the grounds of what would be the hospital compound were buffalo wallows deep in mud and filth. There were several paths running right across the compound and in the back a string of dirty grass huts. The whole area looked miserable. We would have to remake this place completely to build what we were seeking, a nice, neat MEDICO compound.

I outlined to the boys the first essentials: doors on the buildings, cover for the newly arrived gear, the construction of a functioning outhouse, cement for the holes in the walls, patches for the roofs, and ceilings. I told them to emphasize the house first, making it livable, so that from this base they could work on the second building, the hospital. We had dreams of building a third building for a ward, at a later date. They took a deep breath and said, "O.K., sir, the Davis-Rhine Home Construction Gang will go to work. The Lord only knows what will come of it, however." I wasn't worried. I don't think the Lord was, either.

We hiked back to the airport. The plane was unloaded and the pilot was tinkering with the right engine. I said good-by to the boys, climbed into the empty plane, and sat on the floor, looking out of a window. For some reason the plane had to rev up its props for about twenty minutes. Earl and Dwight were sitting on top of the equipment. Sheets of corrugated metal that we had purchased for roofing were flapping in a propwash. It had begun to rain, and they looked forlorn and drenched.

While the pilot held the plane on the end of the landing strip, I kept looking back at these two young men. Here they were, twenty-six and twenty-seven years old, more than half a world away from their wives, out beyond the beyond. They were sitting on a primitive landing strip in an ancient land, just a few miles from the hostile frontier of Red China. When this plane took off, there would be no further transportation into this valley until I returned. Here were two young men who did not speak the native dialect, relying on interpreters whose English was highly inadequate. Here were two very brave young Americans. Suddenly, with a jerk, the plane leaped forward and began its flight up and out of the valley. As the plane flew on, the boys looked like small specks in the distance. They became smaller and smaller. In the months to follow, they became larger and larger.

I spent the next two weeks loading up the military planes from the south and sending them up to the north. I was especially anxious to get a shipment of food off to the boys. They were living off the village market.

My zinc-lined piano was in the warehouse but I did not feel that I could morally send it north on the Lao military aircraft. I went to the commercial airline and asked them if they would fly it up for me. The Frenchmen who ran the airline were so amused at the idea of a piano in the foothills of the Himalayas that they promptly agreed to do it as a contribution to civilization. I took the piano out to the airlines the following day and they shipped it on up to Muong Sing.

I was told a few weeks later that the reaction at Muong Sing was strange. The boys had been eating bizarre native food, and their gastro-intestinal tracts were a bit angry. Each day they thought that the next plane would have canned food aboard it. They went out to the airstrip on this particular day and were positive that good old Dr. Dooley would come through with the food. Instead of the military cargo plane, a commercial plane arrived and unloaded a huge box. They opened it eagerly and found—a piano! Earl said to Dwight, "What can we do with it? We can't play it and we can't eat it." They contemplated just leaving it at the airstrip, but finally they loaded it into an ox-cart and dragged it, strings, hammers, ivories, zinc lining and all, to our newly repaired house.

The boys were doing a lot of construction on the house and the hospital buildings and were getting everything into good shape. Down in the capital I finished handling the formalities with Customs and the government. After I saw that all the essential gear had been shipped up, I flew north again. We would soon be ready to start our hospital work at Muong Sing.

On my arrival, I found that the house was livable and the hospital almost workable.

Our house has three rooms, each about 18 x 23 feet in size. In the center room we put crates up against the wall and covered them with thin mattresses, forming couches on one side and a chair on the other side. The "dining room" table stands in front of one of these couches and some chairs are around its free side. Against one wall, in splendor, stands my piano. On the other side of the door is a bookcase (which has a distinct list to the starboard). We had a very small fireplace which was used as a cooking area until the boys knocked it down; they dug a much larger one and now we boast quite a noble and proud fireplace. One wonders about the need for a fireplace in a tropical land but in this high valley the early morning is quite brisk. At night the cold mist lays low in our valley. Chill enters the night air, but we do not feel it. Warmed by an inner sense of accomplishment we warm ourselves even more by sitting in a semicircle in front of man's most ancient friend, the fire.

The walls of our hut were constructed of a plaster-like substance made of a great deal of mud and a very little cement. The ceiling is high and the floor is stone. Later we laid cement on top of the stone and leveled the floor out so the water did not collect in the middle. Unlike most of the village huts, our house was built on the ground. Many, many months later we put up a corrugated sheet-metal ceiling. This was necessary because the birds collected in our eaves and kept messing up our house, to say nothing of interfering with our meals. The room to the west of the center room is our bedroom. Here we built a platform along the wall and laid five mattresses and bedding rolls on top. Mosquito nets were hung above and we slept Asian style, along one long platform rather than in individual beds. On the top of the platform along each side we built small shelves to keep our clothes in and at the foot of the platform we kept our locker boxes. Along the other wall we had one bed for our rare female guests, and most of our male guests just slept on the platform in Asian style.

The east side of the living room was where our Lao helpers slept, in the same style as ours. They hung more pictures on the whitewashed mud wall than we did. They had more sense. Whereas our wall crumbled when bugs got into the plaster, you could never see what was happening to their wall because it was covered with calendar art.

Staggering along the front of our house was a porch. Where the porch ended in front of the main door, there was an extension covered over and closed in. This became Si's kitchen. We laid a good cement floor, built him a large cooking table upon which he could put his kerosene stoves, and large shelves were built against the wall to store the food.

Back in the corner we built a shower. This was not a shower such as Peter Kessey built in Vang Vieng, ("*la douche du Pierre*"); however, the fundamentals were the same. In Vientiane we had a large 50-gallon tank made with a gooseneck coming out and a shower head on the end of this. This tank was placed on a large flat board connected with lines which went through pulleys and came down near the other side of the kitchen. We could lower this huge tank of water through the system of pulleys to easy filling-level, and dump buckets of heated water from the well into the tank. Then the tank would be pulled up by the lines until it was about eight feet high. We hung a piece of tarpaulin for a shower curtain, built a drainage pit and a bamboo floor as the shower deck, and enjoyed all the comforts of a hot-shower-at-home.

Out in the back we built an outhouse in magnificent style. While I was away on a village trip one day, the boys painted over its door, "Uncle Tom's Cabin." On the inside of the door facing the seat, I put up a large piece of paper with all the Lao alphabet on it so that we could learn the script in our leisure moments.

On the front porch we built a shaving area consisting of nothing but a wooden board with two circle holes cut into it and enameled basins countersunk into these holes. Underneath the basins we put a metal drain joining a rubber tube which then ran into the ground. Under the ground the boys planted some large green bamboo pipes which drained out into a ditch in front of the compound. Quite an ingenious Asian water system. On the side of this washing area was another large 55-gallon water barrel made out of an empty gasoline drum. This was kept filled from the well.

The well? This was a personal gift of Ambassador Horace Smith. Within a few weeks after we arrived, Ambassador Smith came to visit us. This was an extremely nice gesture. Never before, when I was in Laos, did any high American dignitary ever visit me. We were tremendously thrilled that he came. He said, "Tom, what can I specifically give to you?" I said, "Sir, two wells and a jeep." He laughed and asked me to explain myself. I pointed out that we wanted to build a cement well and that cement was heavy, therefore costly, I did not want to be so expensive to the Lao Ministry of Health so early. And I wished to transport my jeep to the north. This too was a heavy problem in transportation. Both of these were "luxuries," because we really could get our water from the local river and walk instead of ride in a jeep. The Ambassador said he would take care of it and within three days the Embassy plane returned bringing us a jeep and the cement rings for two wells.

There is a story about the jeep. Muong Sing has one "road" that runs the length of our valley. I use the word road in quotation marks advisedly because this road, which runs about 20 miles, is a single buffalo-cart lane. No other type of vehicle had been used on this road until the Army brought a jeep up and, a few months later, we received our jeep. In all of northern Laos, for hundreds of square miles, there were only two jeeps and only twenty miles of "road."

Nevertheless, one day a few months later, these two jeeps actually ran into each other.

We loved to put titles on things and after the well was completed and a little well-house above it, we tried for weeks to think of an appropriate title. "Smith's Water Hole" sounded a little fresh for three young men to use in honor of an Ambassador. "American-Nam," meaning American water, sounded a bit too nationalistic. Ambassador Smith's name does not lend itself to rhyme and so his well remained unnamed but not unappreciated.

The Laos Minister of Public Works sent us an old carpenter friend from Nam Tha to help us build our buildings. We called him "Bolum," which means "uncle." Bolum didn't believe in any of this modern stuff, like nails or gasoline-run buzz saws; everything had to be wedged and cut by hand. It took Bolum quite some time to get these done, but never can we complain of architectural shoddiness. Our buildings certainly do not look as though they were built in haste. We asked him to build a small roof over the well house and he ended up building something massive enough to be a pagoda.

Every little thing is a problem in Laos. To make a building you have to chop the tree down, skin the bark off of it, cut it into planks, then cut the planks to fit and then groove and wedge and paint. Nothing is easy in the primeval forest, as we knew when we came to Asia.

Since Chai was now a married man, we had to build a house for him on the back of the compound. The poor boys needed Chai very badly during the opening months, but Chai had come down with a case of yellow jaundice. He spent his first three weeks in Muong Sing as the first patient in our new hospital. When his house was finished, he moved into it.

Once in Nam Tha I had a patient whose leg had been hideously bloated by infection and then withered up. There are pictures of this boy, named Owi, in my book *The Edge of Tomorrow.* When Owi heard that I had returned to Muong Sing, a full day's walk from Nam Tha, he came to me to join our team. We were delighted to hire him, as he is a very bright boy. He became the assistant to Si. When Owi had to have an assistant he found La, a Thai Lu tribe boy, to help him. Therefore the staff of the house consisted of Si, Owi and La—Owi, a Thai Dam tribe boy; La, a Thai Lu; Si, a Lao, each speaking a dialect a little different. Each of them had their own small specialization (not unlike the American Medical Association). Face is tremendously important in the Orient. I would offend Si if I went directly to Owi to ask for something. Si had given to Owi responsibility for the grounds and for the food contributed by the patients as payment in the clinic. Owi had given La responsibility for the house—cleaning, dusting, and making of the beds. The two boys helped serve dinner while Si, who had previously cooked the dinner, would sit down at the table and eat with us.

This division of authority is important, and we would always go to Si to have him tell La and Owi to do various things. Owi had a battalion of small kids from the village who assisted him. When the lawn had too much debris on it, when the water buffaloes had gotten in and made a wallow somewhere, when a bad wind had broken a lot of palm trees and their fronds were all over the ground, Owi would call his battalion together and they would sweep over the compound, cleaning it much as hordes of locusts clean a field of corn.

As none of us believe in exploitation, these children were paid for their work. They were paid by being allowed to pick out some jewelry from the huge chest of costume jewelry that had been collected for us by children all around America. The children of our village would come and say to Owi, "Do you have some work for us?" What this really meant was, "May we have a piece of costume jewelry?" They knew us well enough to know that we "gave" nothing away, and that they must earn these things. It appealed to their pride and we felt this was important.

On the same theory we demanded that all of our patients pay us to the best of their ability. They cannot pay in money but they can pay in kind. An operation would cost several chickens. A delivery, one chicken. Pills would cost eggs or rice or fruit. When the pineapple season came, we would get as many as twenty or thirty pineapples at the end of the day's sick call. We needed this food, we had a staff of some ten or fifteen to feed, and a hospital full of patients; we put all of the donated food to good use. I think that easy and condescending charity robs people, and perhaps nations, of their self-respect.

Once the clinic began to run, it became important that we find a student staff. I was not too concerned with the training of Earl and Dwight myself. I am not interested alone in the amount of antibiotics that circulate in the bodies of our patients. But I am most interested in the amount of education that circulates in the hearts and minds of the people of our high valley. After our departure this will last longer than will their blood level of penicillin.

Therefore, we needed to find students and begin our training program. We went to the Military Commandant and suggested to him that we open a training school for the military. He was delighted and said that he would have some men sent over to us the next day. The next day ten men came and never have I seen such a motley crew. (I suppose my professor at St. Louis University Medical School said the same thing after he met his new freshman class.) The Lao army students were made up of several tribes, the Thai Dam, Thai Lu, Yao and Lao. Each tribe considers the others just a little bit inferior.

My first glance at the students made one boy almost an immediate favorite. His name was Deng. Deng was very short and looked about fourteen, although he claimed to be twenty-one. He was very olive-skinned, with a dark heavy shank of hair and two of the widest doe eyes I have ever seen. Months later as he would see surgery, see medical miracles, see the progress of patients, his eyes would get bigger and bigger. It looked as though his whole face were engulfed by the whites of his eyes. Deng stayed on with us while other students came and went. Deng became a very intricate part of the Dooley team at Muong Sing. We all grew to love him very much. He became a competent compassionate corpsman.

The first thing we had to do was to explain to students that they must not pick their noses. There were a few other commandments, such as:

"Thou shalt not spit on the deck.

"Thou shalt not scratch thyself.

"When thou wearest rubber gloves, thou shalt not shake hands with thy friend.

"Thou shalt not toss the left-over water on the floor.

"Thou shalt not open capsules and dump powder in hand of patient, but thou shalt push pill in mouth of patient.

"Thou shalt cut thy fingernails to the quick, including the fifth fingernail.

"Thou *shalt* and thou *shalt not* one thousand times."

The next step was to try to get them to be a little better group of men. The first thing this entailed was teeth cleaning. Earl, who had a penchant for dentistry, began to scrape the tartar off their teeth, and for their first pay we gave them toothbrushes and toothpaste. We introduced our student staff to the bizarre habit of daily toothbrushing.

Then we had to reteach ourselves that patience is the companion of wisdom.

As the months went on we grew more and more fond of these boys. Later we brought three girls into study with us. However, the same problems that arise in coeducational schools began to arise in our hospital. A little pinching here and there, a little play here and there, and a slight deterioration of the work level.

People talk about the differences between Americans and the Asians. It is obvious that there are differences, but these are good. We have no desire in Laos to build a mirror image of an American hospital. We have no desire that my staff mimic the staff of anybody else anywhere. We just want to illustrate to these people what we are, and if they wish to adopt our system, fine. If they do not, then though we believe it's their loss, it is their decision to make.

Differences of race and culture are not accurate measurements of superiority or inferiority. As I see it, uniformity is something to be abhorred. The world would be a very unattractive place if everything conformed. China through her commune system is trying to build such conformity. It is not a pleasant thought, because it is an offense against freedom.

The great richness of our universe is due above all to its diversity. We should take honorable pride in the distinct accomplishments of the Irish, the French, the Asian, the Negro. We must be equally aware that the accomplishments of others are proper subjects for their pride too. These thoughts were present in each day's work. These differences were obvious and pleasing to us.

Our students pitched into each day's work with a wonderful vitality. They soon grew to have no fear of us. They came to our house in the morning and mixed their own coffee, sat around and read magazines (looking at the pictures), and were very much members of the team, not employees of a Westerner. Some things were hard for them. I imagine that we three Americans made an appalling sight: we talked so fast, we walked so fast, we did such bizarre things. It must have been more difficult for them to adjust to us than it was for us to adjust to them. The instinctive pride that these young men and women had in becoming members of our team was a very bright and precious thing. We had to care for that pride and nurture it. We had to take their abilities and their youthfulness and teach them to grow tall and straight, glowing and strong.

There was much they had not seen of raw life even in their own Asian land. The sick and the wretched often live and die in the corners of their huts, out of the sight of other villagers. Suddenly our student staff were slapped with all the drudgery and frustration of medical work. They knew some of the hopelessness, and the unremitting, grinding treadmill of work. They saw that the sick vomit, the dying die, the maimed limp forever. We had to show our students that along with the ugly part of life they would also see that precious thing called hope. Just as the rain forest trees soar over even our mountaintops, these young men must soar over the heads of their compatriots.

I treated these men as I treated my own two Americans. To an outsider one would notice little difference in the way I spoke to or dealt with any of them. This is as Earl and Dwight would have wished it, and it was essential for our students. I am their brother, yes, but their older brother. Though Asians seldom speak roughly to each other, I frequently spoke strongly to my students. Once when Deng, for about the forty-fifth time, had put an instrument back into the case unwashed, I blew my stack. In front of several of his student friends, I told him that he was not a capable man and that I had no room in my hospital for men who did not do things as I told them. I told Deng to go. I would replace him with someone else. I know I spoke to him very sternly but this had been an offense committed too many times. Deng slunk outside and cried his eyes red. Several hours later he came back and pleaded, "*Kho tot kenoi, Thanh Mo America, dai.* I'm sorry, Doctor America, please. . . ." Of course he was forgiven and has never put an unclean instrument away since that time.

It is a very wonderful thing to watch the young men grow and mature. It was feeling the pulse of existence in our high valley. They watched people dying, suffering, being healed, being born. Our working together in the languid afternoon, hiking together down mountain trails, our shooting the rapids on boats, gave us a common touch of humanity and made it evident that the brotherhood of man exists as surely as does the Fatherhood of God.

Asians respond to the help of brotherhood with affection. With these men of Asia I found my life's work. My convictions have gained in strength whatever, from time to time, they may have lost in disillusion. I will work amongst these people. I will train them as best I can. But I must do more than just treat the sick. I must bear witness, I must speak up as often as possible and according to my ability. I must tell other Americans of these Asians. I think all men should reaffirm what they know, what they believe. I want to speak of the spirit of Asia.

The spirit of man is not a nebulous thing. The spirit of man is this palpable thing in the hearts of Deng and Chai, Earl and Dwight. On this earth each man must find his field of work. For Tom Dooley the workbench is Asia. Here where the mountains mingle with the night, where there is the anguish of living and dying, here in these high valleys I will work for all my days.

A few weeks after our arrival in Muong Sing a man came to our still unfinished house, with a huge basket of flowers and fruits. He wanted to perform a *baci.* When we first arrived in Nam Tha in 1957, there was a certain hostility and coldness amongst the people of the valley. We were new, we were white men who had strange techniques, we did strange things. They had never seen us before, and they had heard much from the Communists and from the jungle rulers, both good and bad. The situation was not the same when we arrived in Muong Sing. The word of our work in Nam Tha in the preceding years had spread, and this man's visit was proof.

The traditional ceremony of *baci* consists of tying the white cotton string of friendship around the wrists of those to whom the *baci* is offered. As each string is tied, one makes the wish, "I wish you happiness," "I wish you longevity," "I wish you much love," "I wish you wives and many children," "I wish you blue skies, bright night and good health."

We did not know why these people had come to us to offer us a *baci,* as we had yet to treat them. The man brought his wife, sister, aunt, uncle and a half a dozen children. We talked about many things, always trying to figure out exactly why he was offering this *baci* for us. Then he pulled over his little son, yanked down his pants and showed me a neat hairline scar. I had done a herniorrhaphy on the boy in 1957. He remembered us well and was grateful for our returning to North Laos. I remembered that when his son had been my patient they had walked all the way across the mountain that separates Muong Sing from Nam Tha. Now I live on his side of that mountain.

With men like him speaking in our behalf it took no time at all before we were a most accepted group in town. Within a few weeks people didn't even notice us in the market place. This was a pleasant thing. We wanted to become an intimate and integral part of the community life of the villagers. We had indeed with these people of the valley, but we wondered about the people of the mountain.

Good fortune shone on us. Only a few days after our arrival, a young man was brought to us whose face had been hideously mauled by a bear. This lad belonged to the high mountain tribe called the Kha Kho. The boy had a filthy wound and a huge hole in the cheek. You could shove two fingers into a yawning, foul-smelling wound just below the eye and the fingers poked out of the roof of his mouth. This pus-filled hole had been stuffed with tobacco and monkey fur. His right eye was torn loose and many of his teeth were broken. The whole upper jawbone was fractured in several places.

We had to do a series of operations on him, first removing the loosened maxillary plate. It took us several days of cleaning him up with antibiotics and daily washings in order to find what tissue was worth saving. We had to remove what was left of his lacerated eyeball. Then under general anesthesia we were able to loosen the good skin from around the jaw, the eye, the side of the nose, and the cheekbone. Without tension we pulled good tissue over and closed up the hole in his face. It healed well, leaving only a jagged scar. Though to us this still looked awful, to him it was a near miracle. From a miserable youngster with a horribly dirty, foul face, this lad had become quite an acceptable sight. We discharged him from the hospital but he returned in a few days with a very small dog. He got on his knees and held this dog up to us as an offering of gratitude. I smiled at him and said "*Cup Chai*," and added, "*Het menh yanh.* What can I do with it?" The boy looked at me in surprise and responded, "Eat it." We were adopted into the Kha Kho family of men.

Many people became our friends. So did this little dog. Dwight named him Fang because he was so utterly harmless and cowardly. All of the children in our area called the dog Fang too. Occasionally Dwight would get angry, growl at the dog and say, "Come here, Fang, son of Claw." When the Asians would try to repeat that, the sound that came out was unprintable in Lao or English.

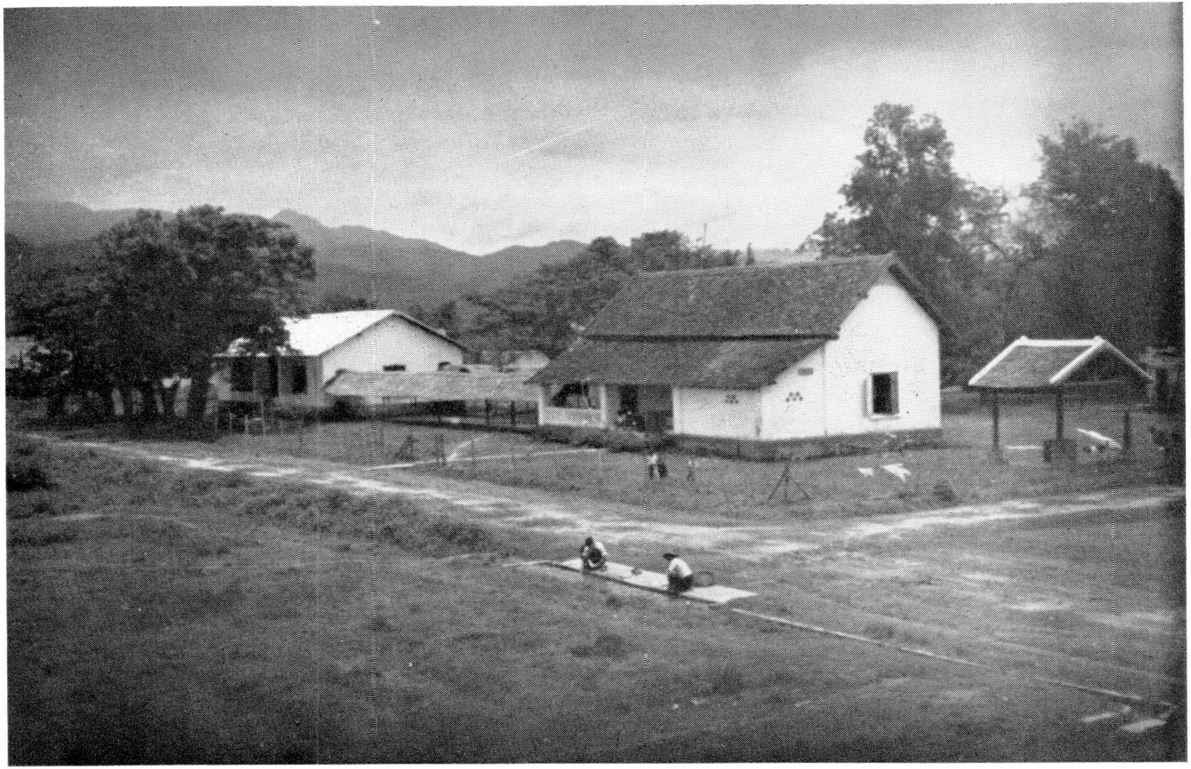

My favorite picture: our house and clinic in Muong Sing.
In the background a storm is gathering over Red China.

The daily sick-call line.

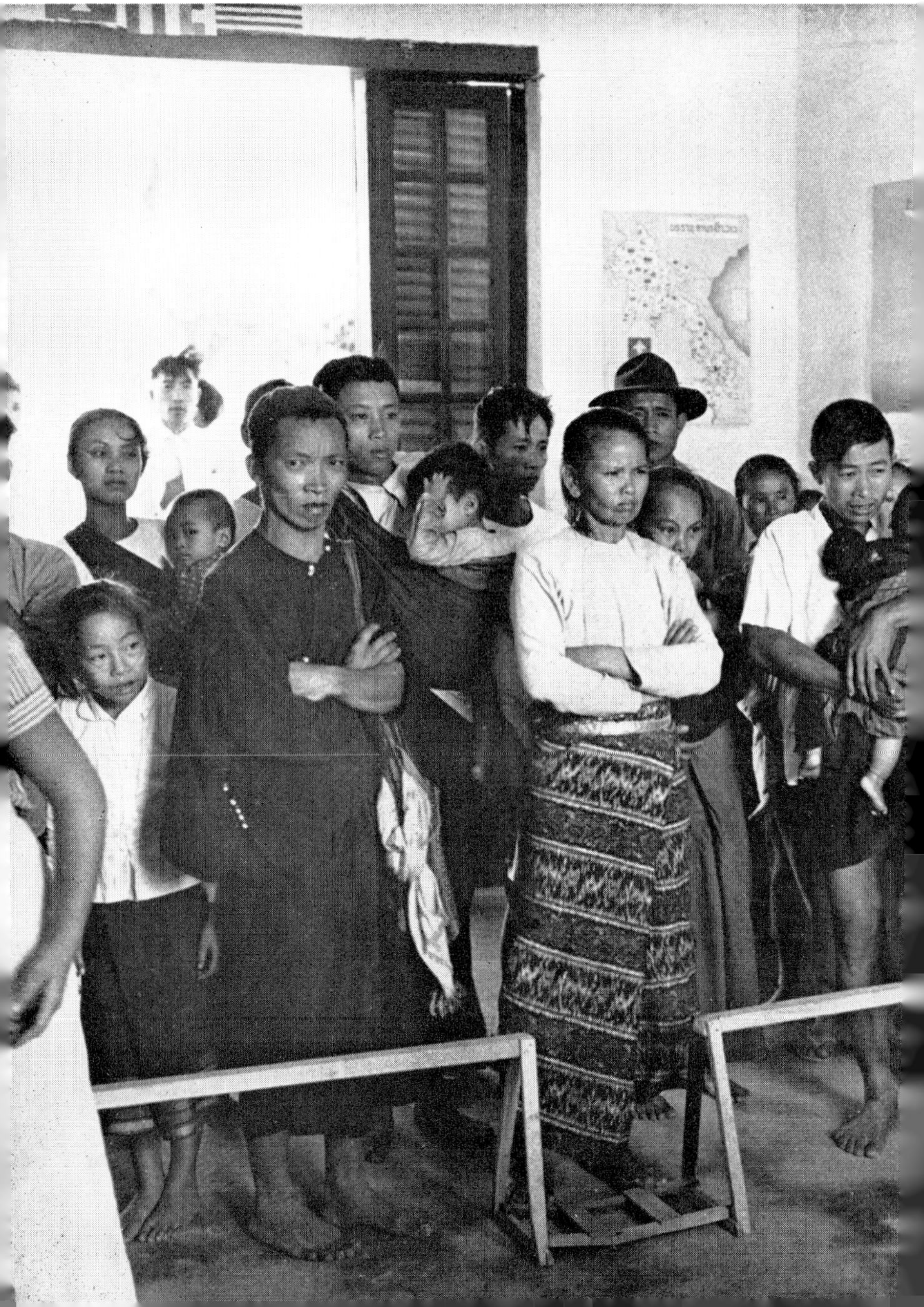

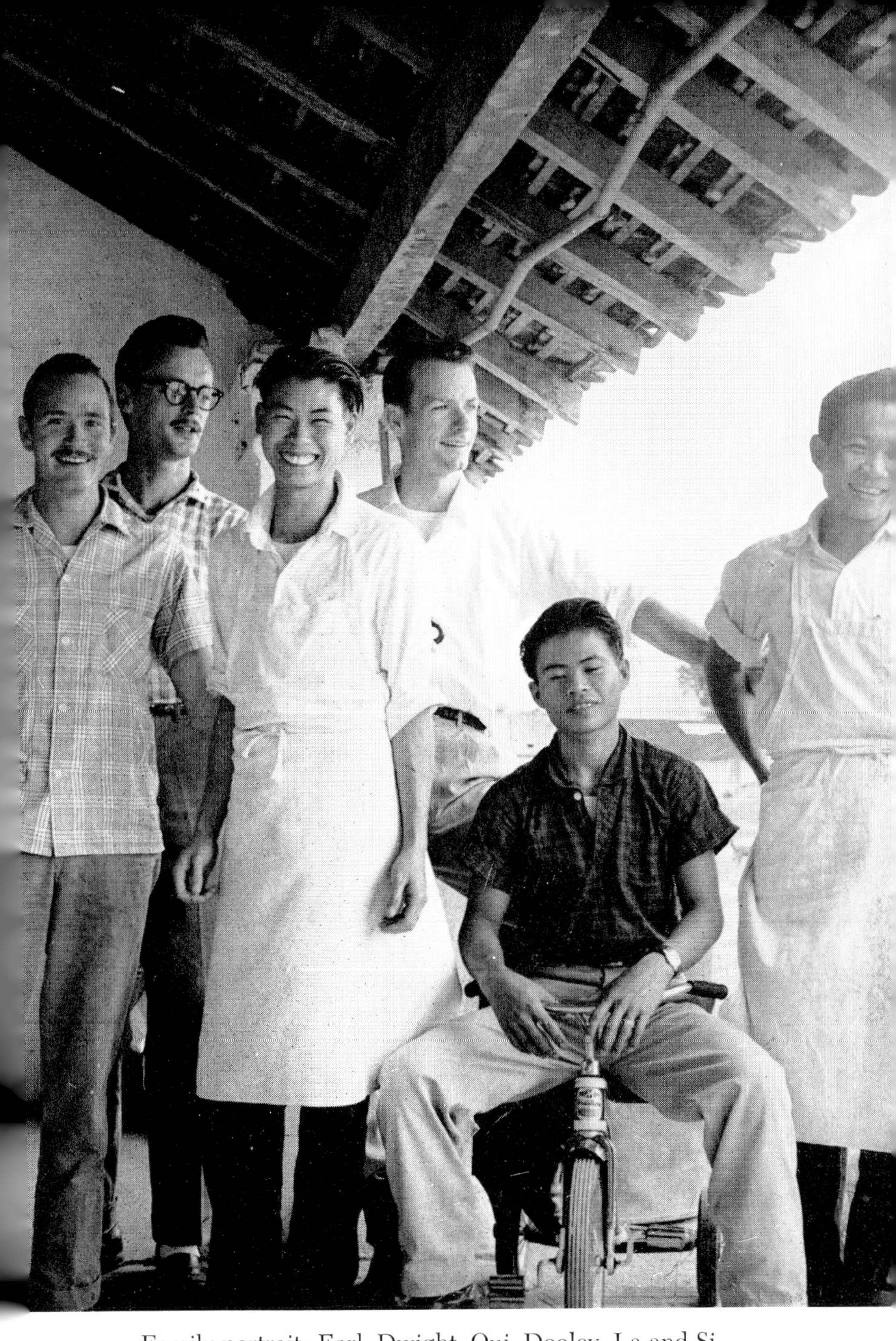

Family portrait: Earl, Dwight, Oui, Dooley, La and Si.

The doctor's post of honor in the clinic.

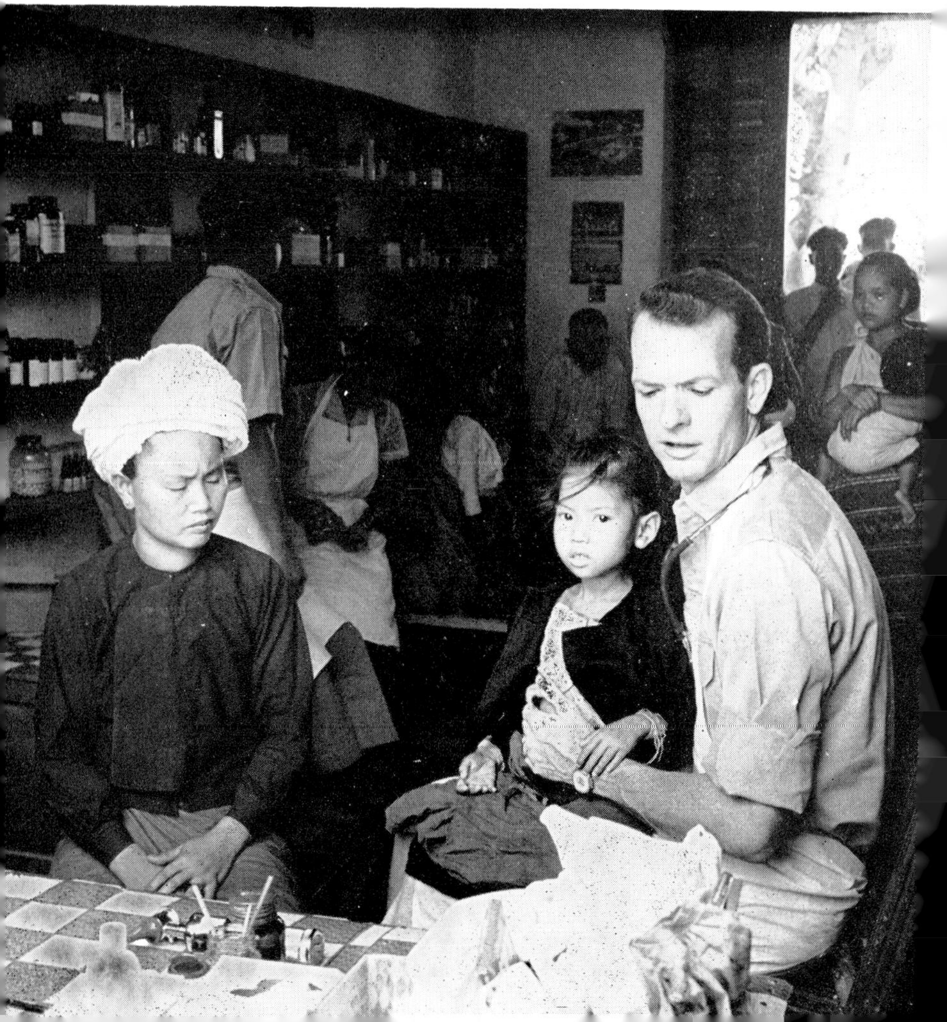

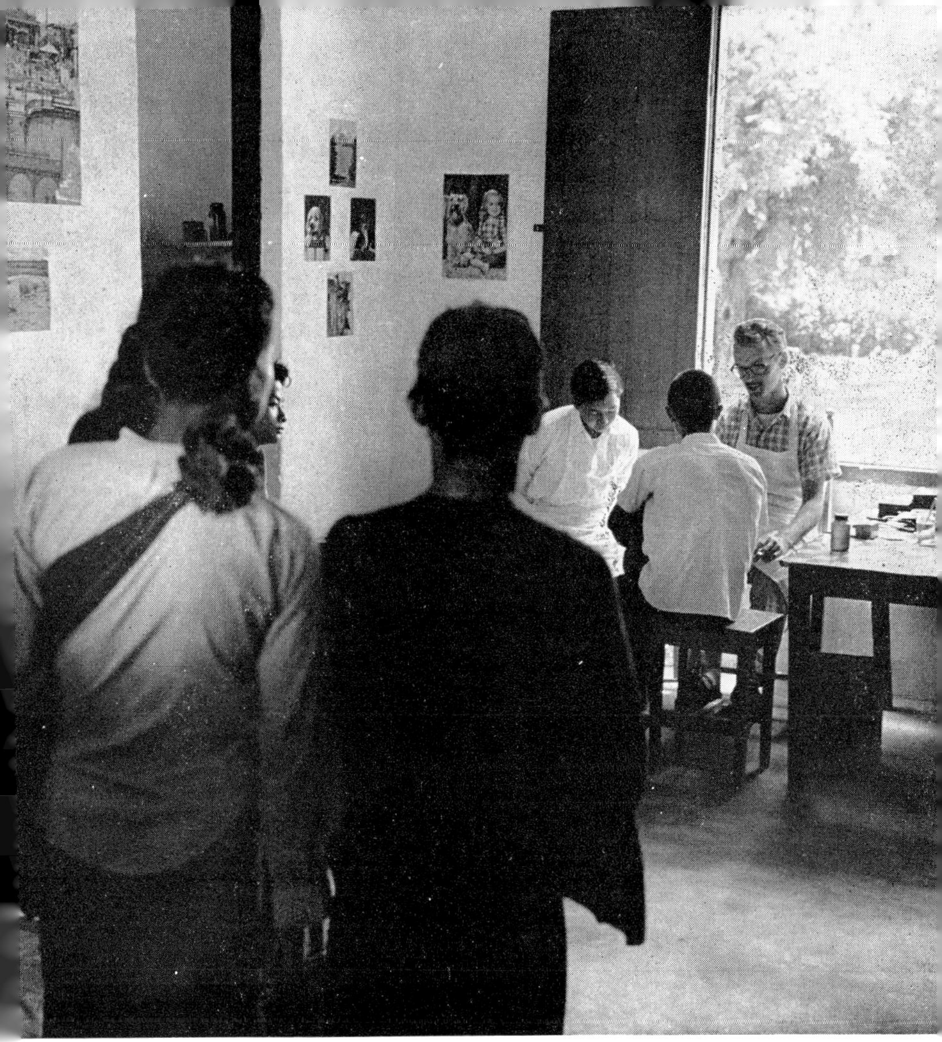

Dwight Davis takes the clinic line.

Doctor Schweitzer calls this a "confab."

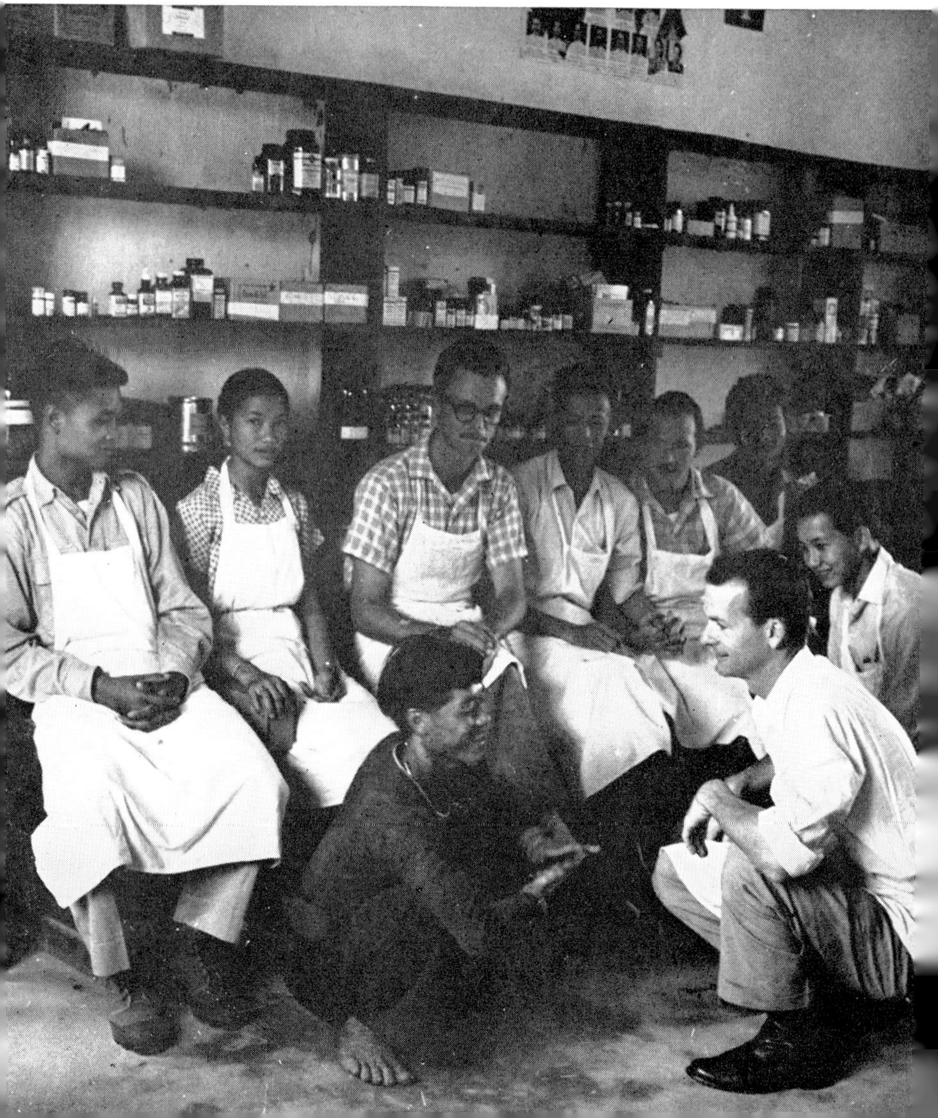

Surgery.

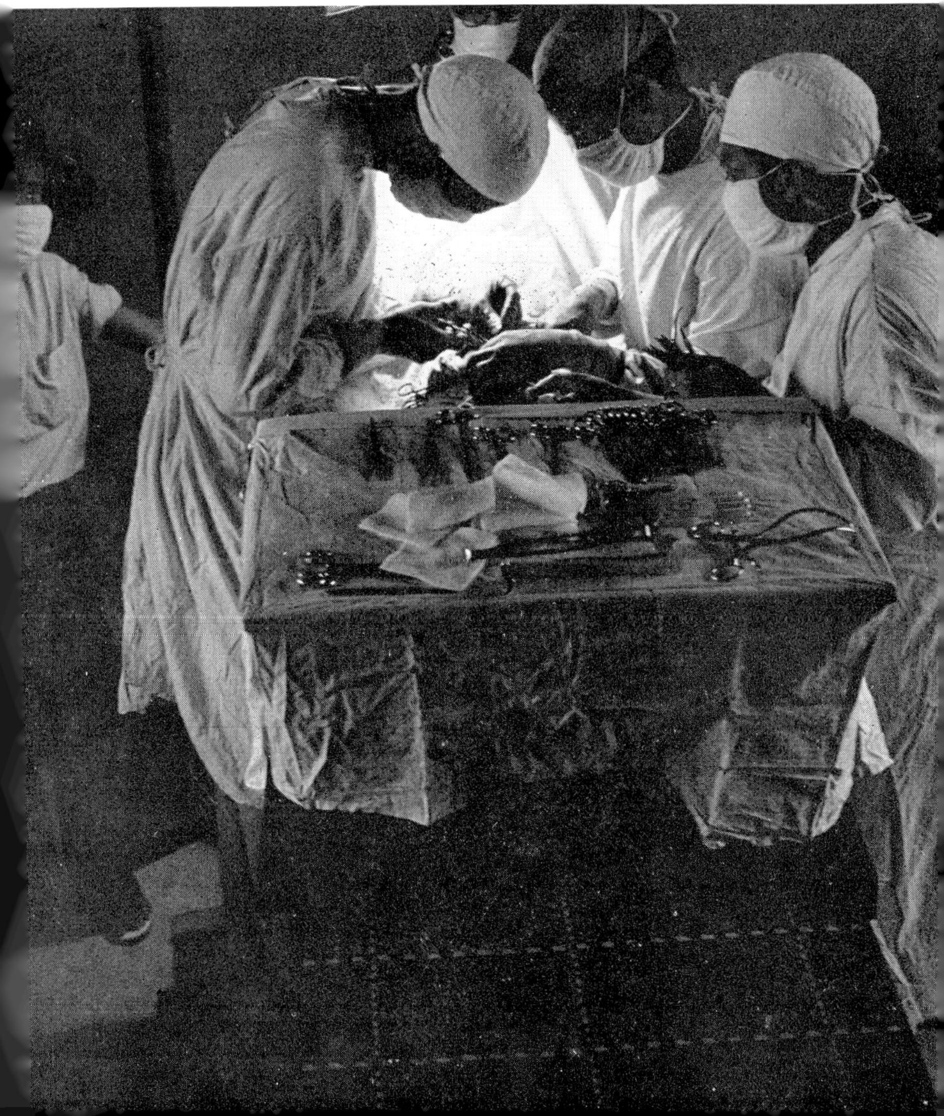

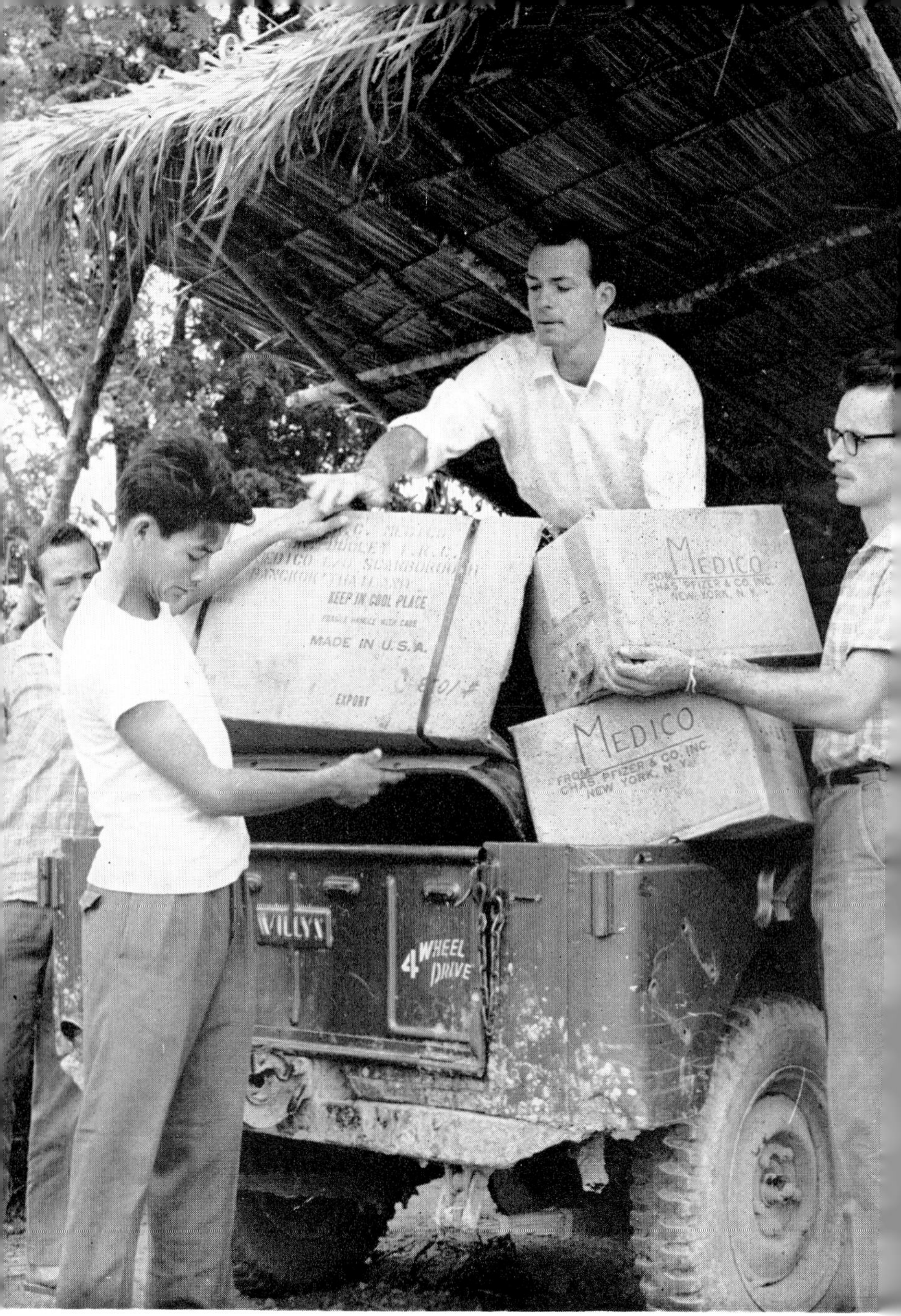

Earl, Chai, Dooley and Dwight unload newly-arrived drugs, the gift of Pfizer.

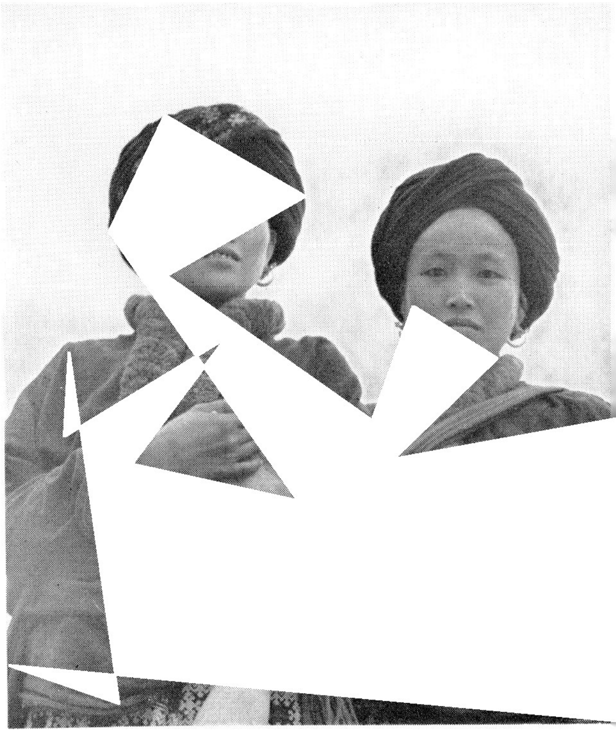

Two Lao debutantes drop in for a visit—and so do two generations, grandmother and grandchild.

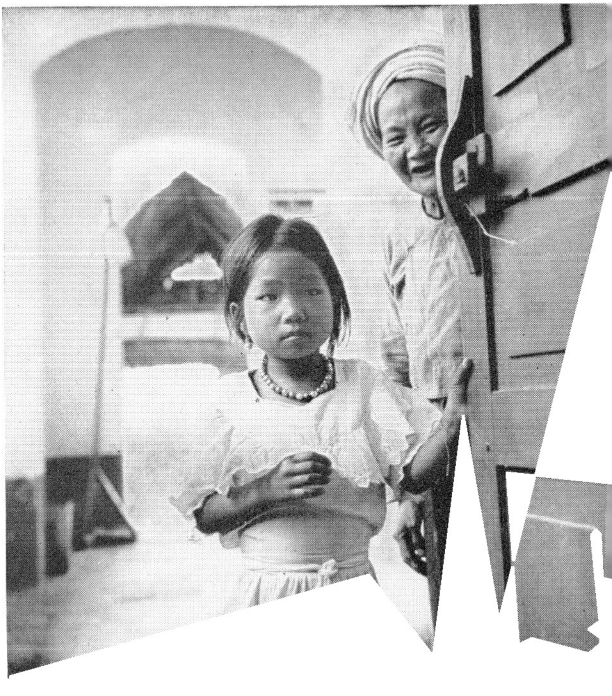

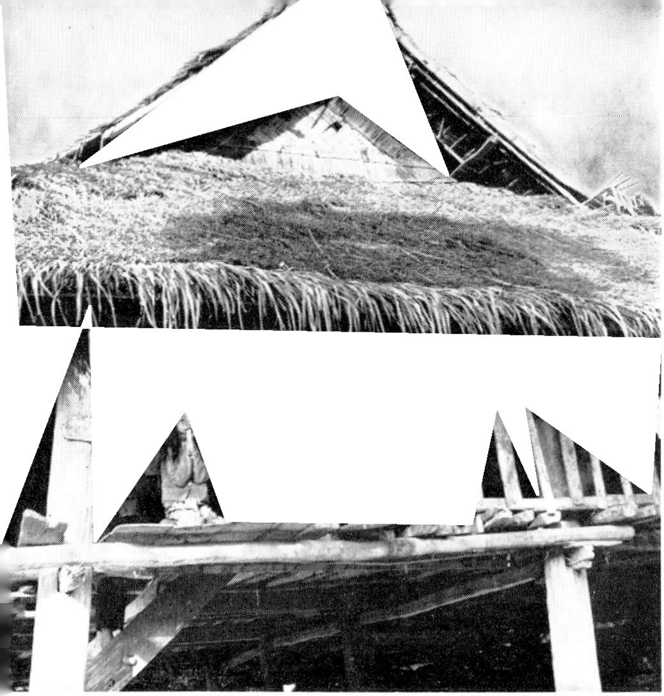

Little girls are the same the world over—and so are little boys, even young Buddhist monks.

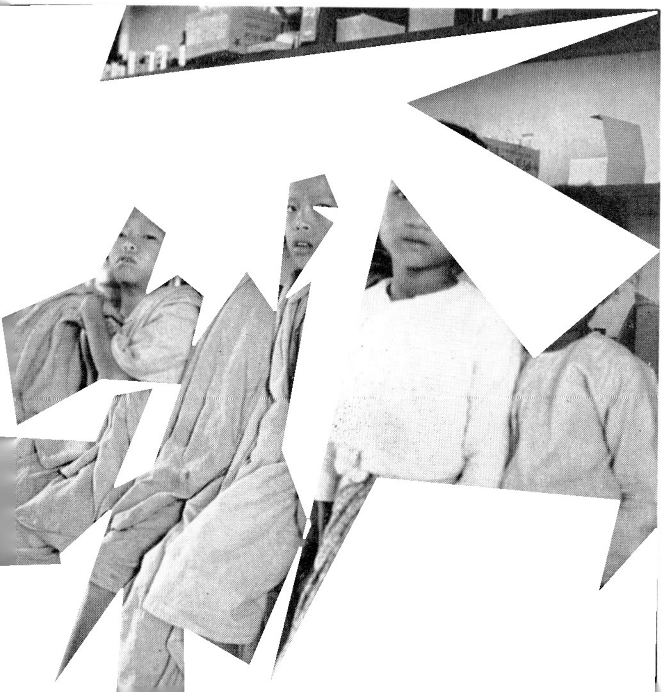

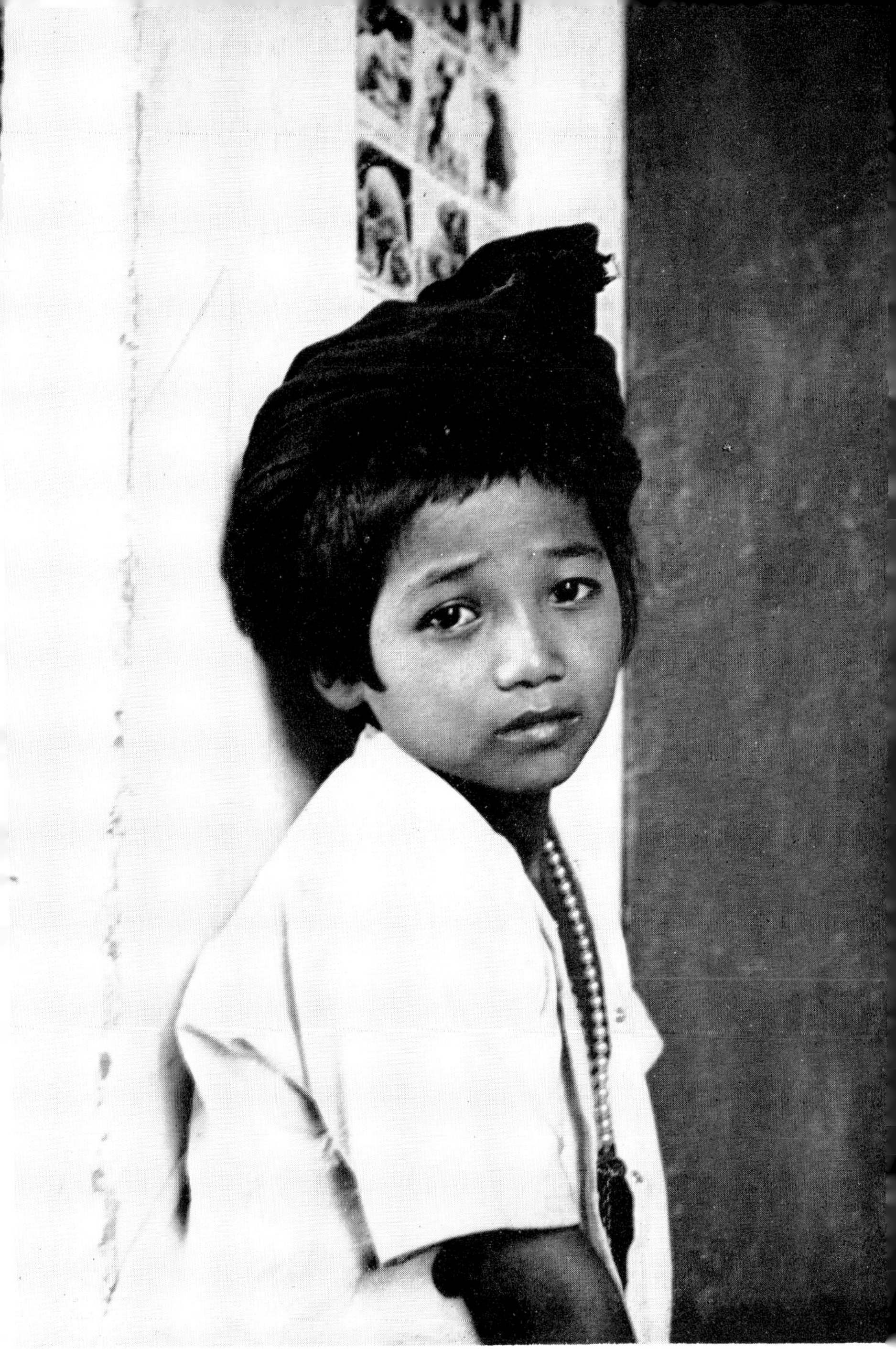

"Will you help MEDICO to help Dr. Dooley to help me and my people to learn to help ourselves?"

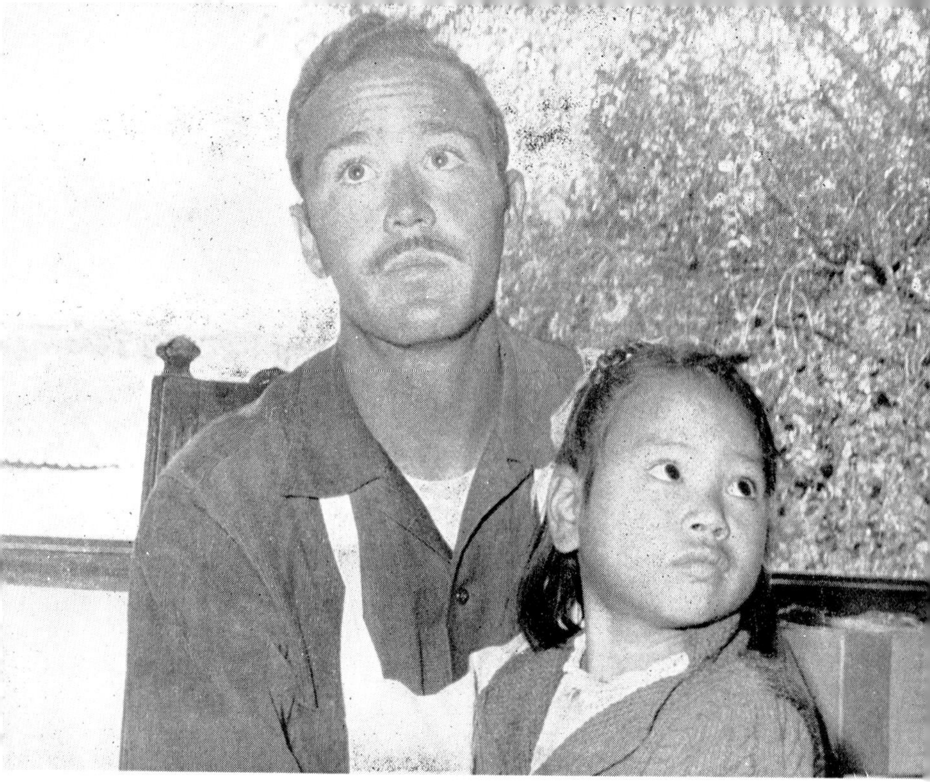

Earl Rhine and his daily visitor (see Chapter 6).

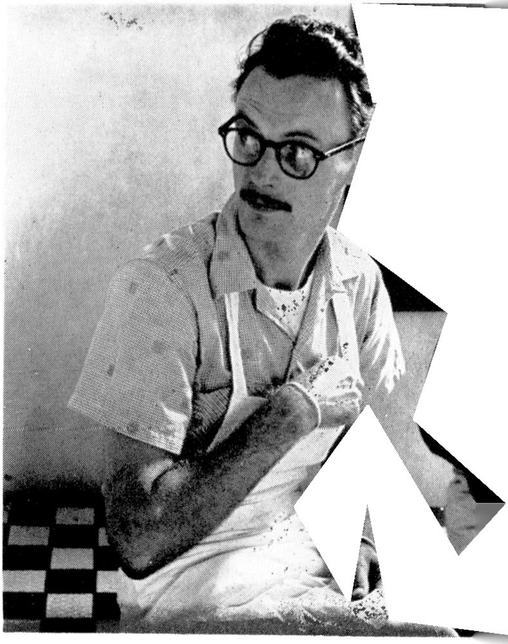

Dwight Davis wearing Lao white cotton strings binding our nations together.

The brush isn't too good, but the toothpaste tastes fine.

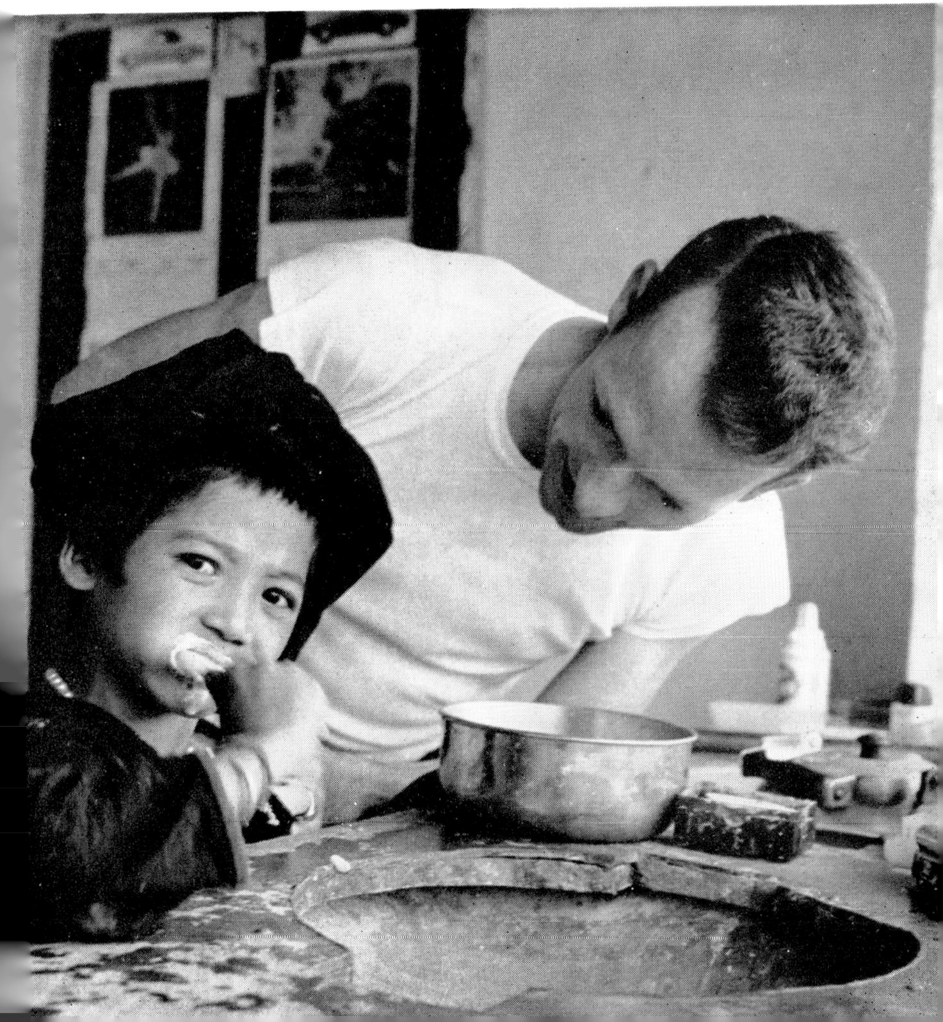

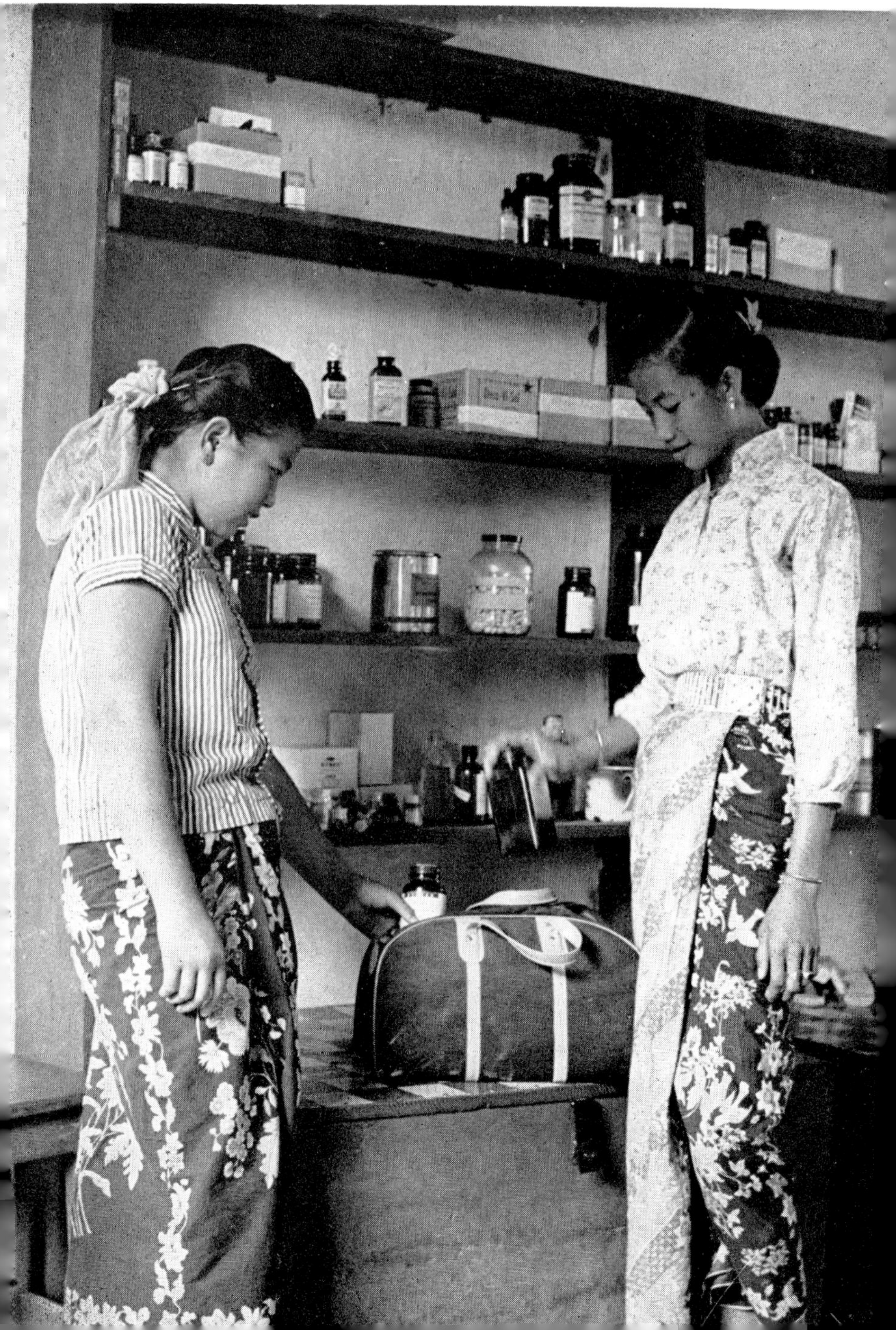

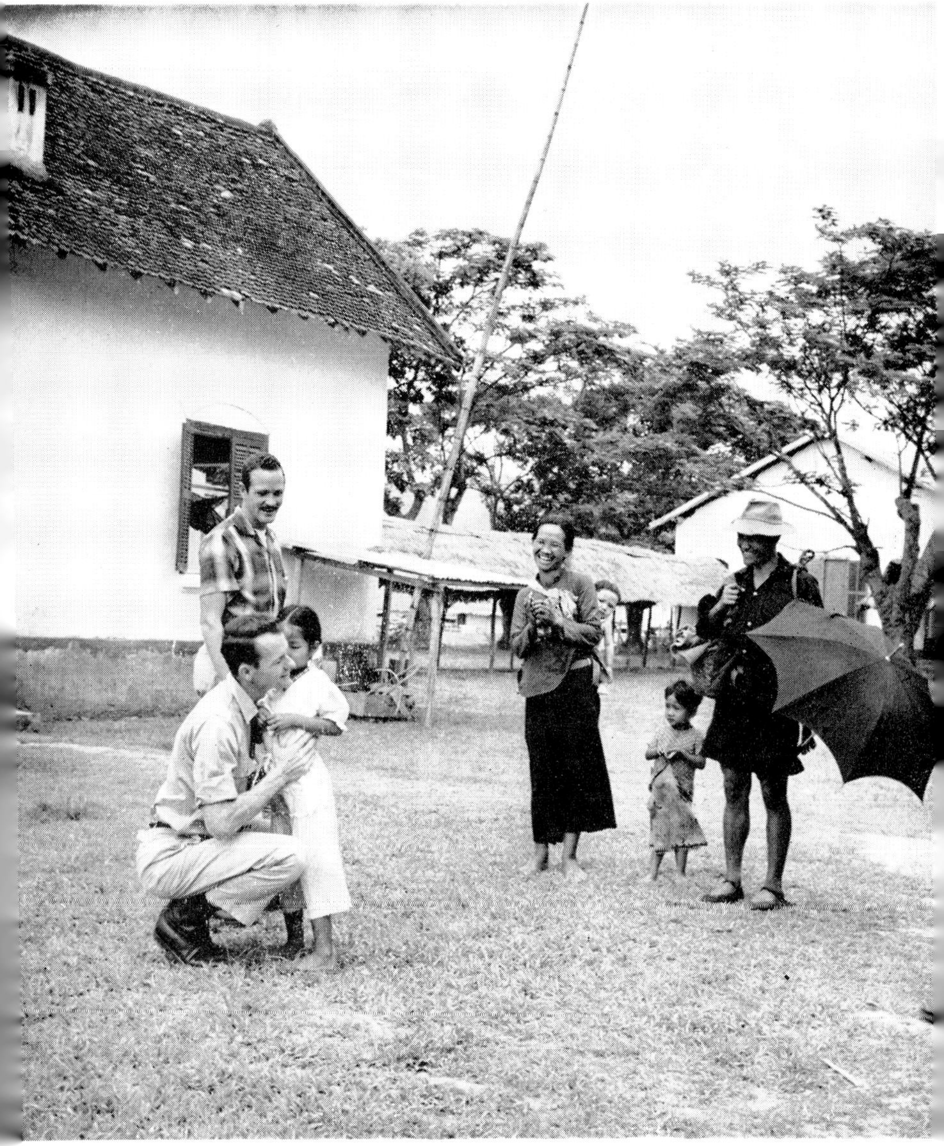

A family scene in our backyard.

Left: Changtip and Oula refilling their midwife-kit.

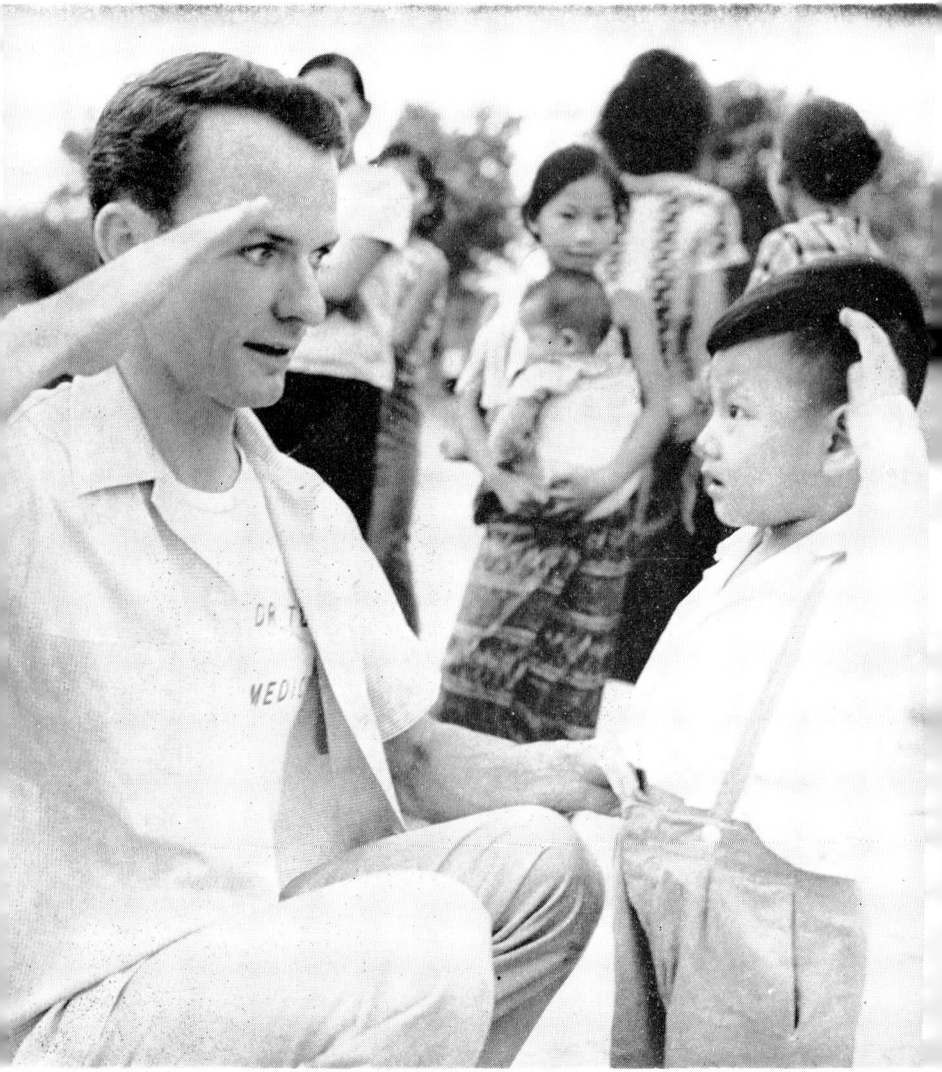

Who outranks who?

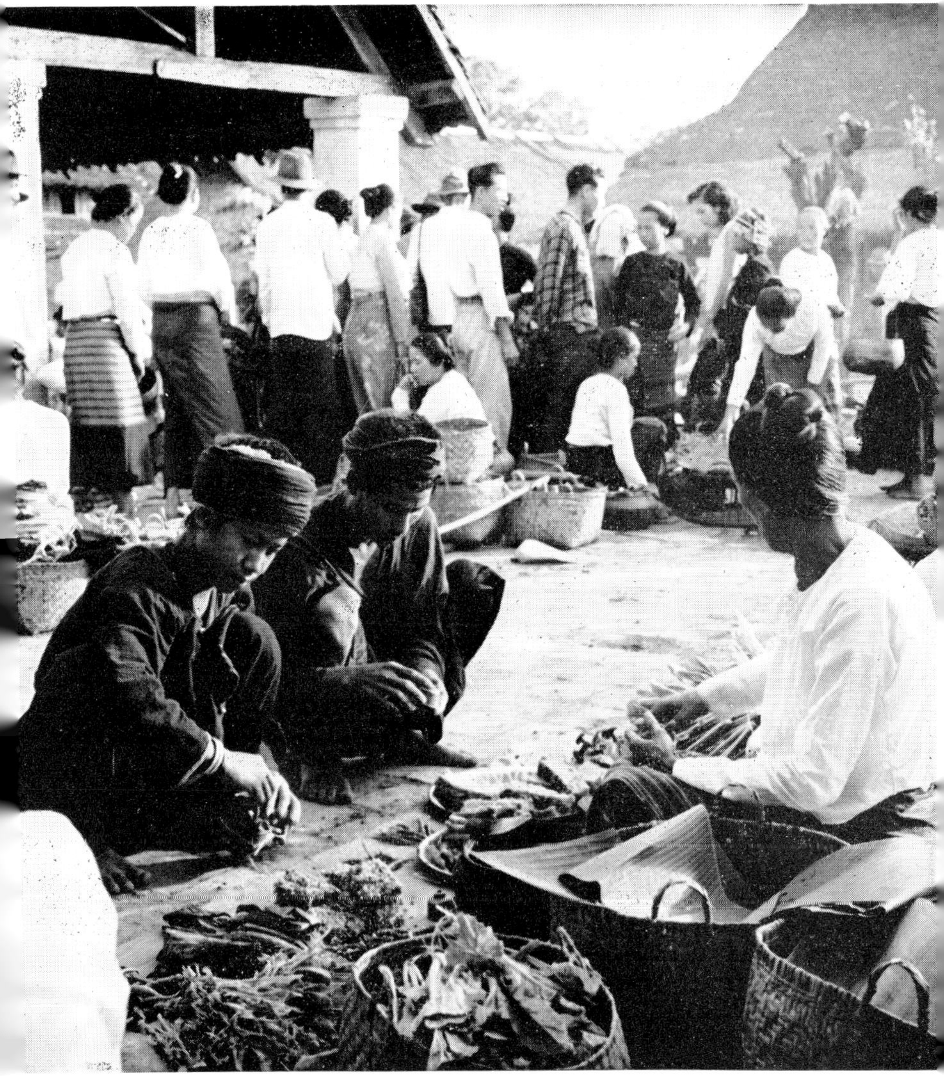

The village market.

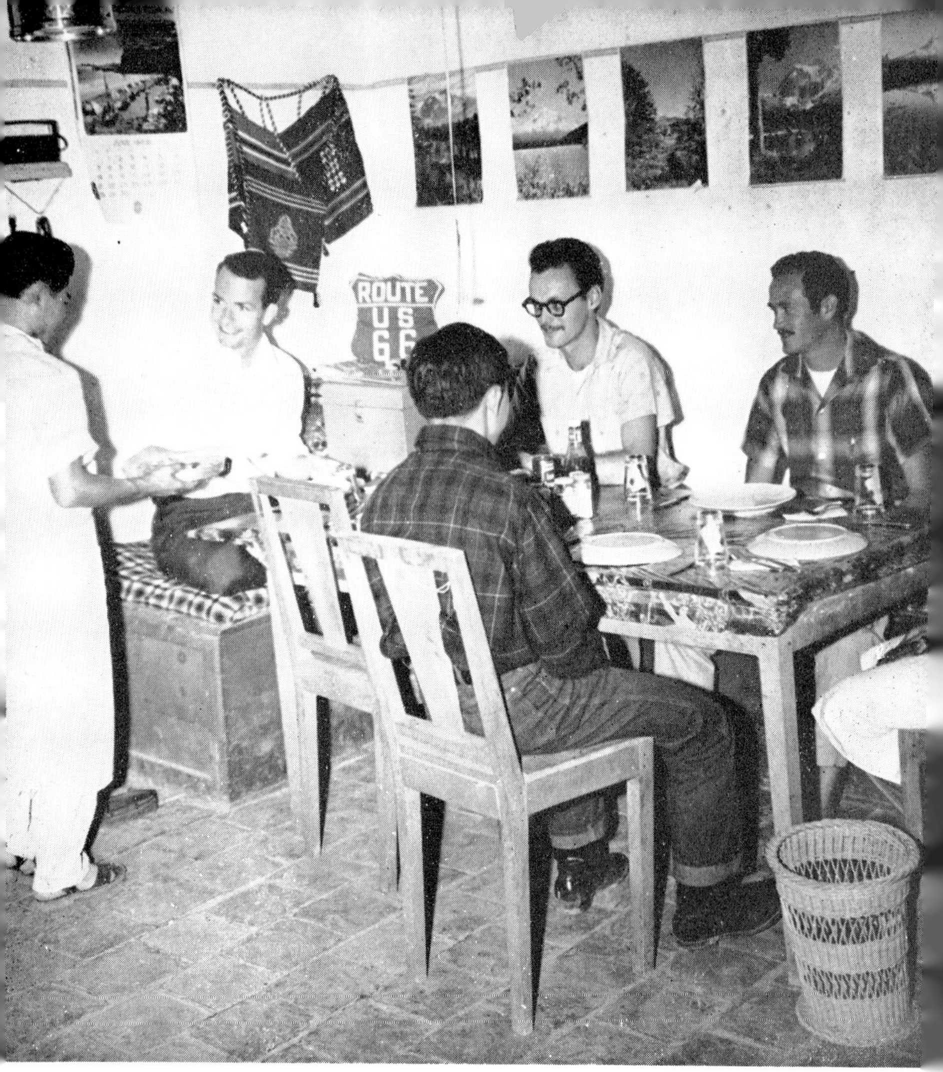

Family dinner: three languages, three races, one love.

A Mao tribesman, wasting away. He was floated down the river from Red China.

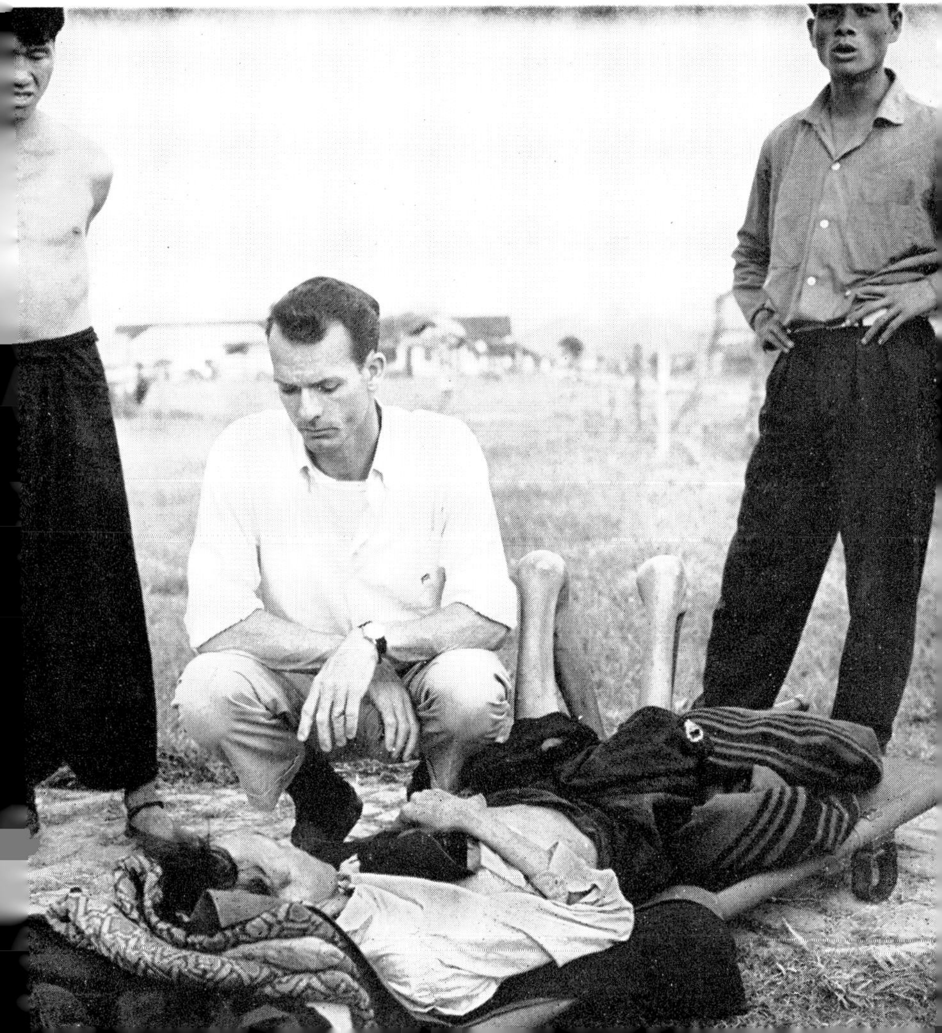

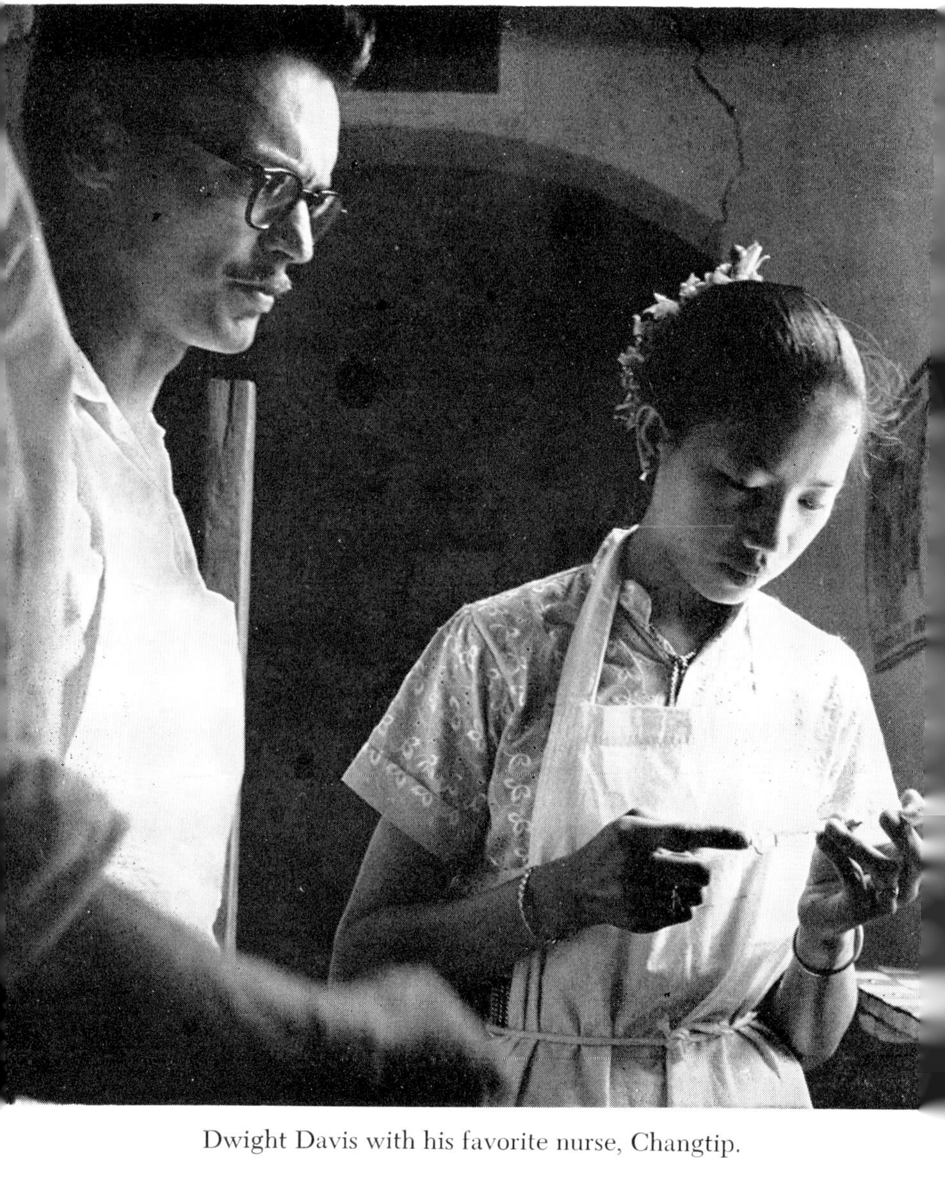

Dwight Davis with his favorite nurse, Changtip.

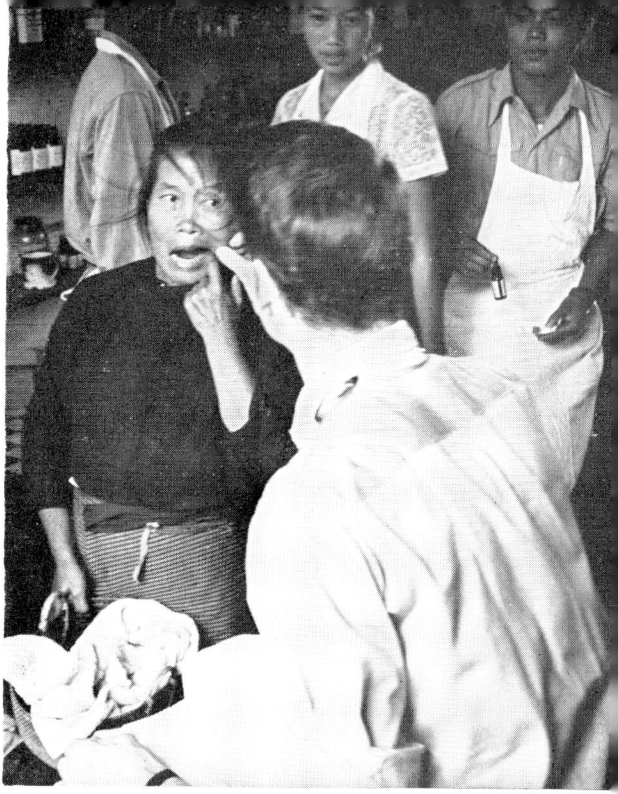

"It's this tooth, doctor."

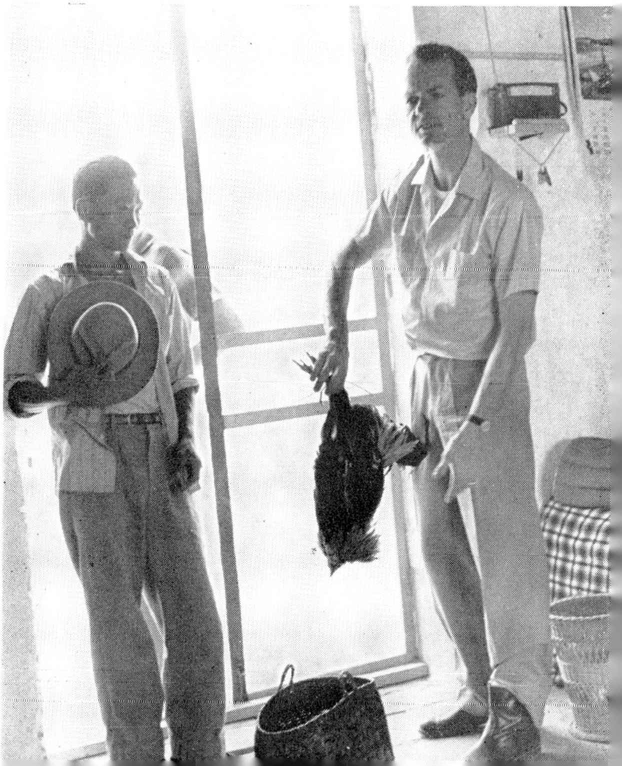

A proud father makes payment for delivery of his first-born son.

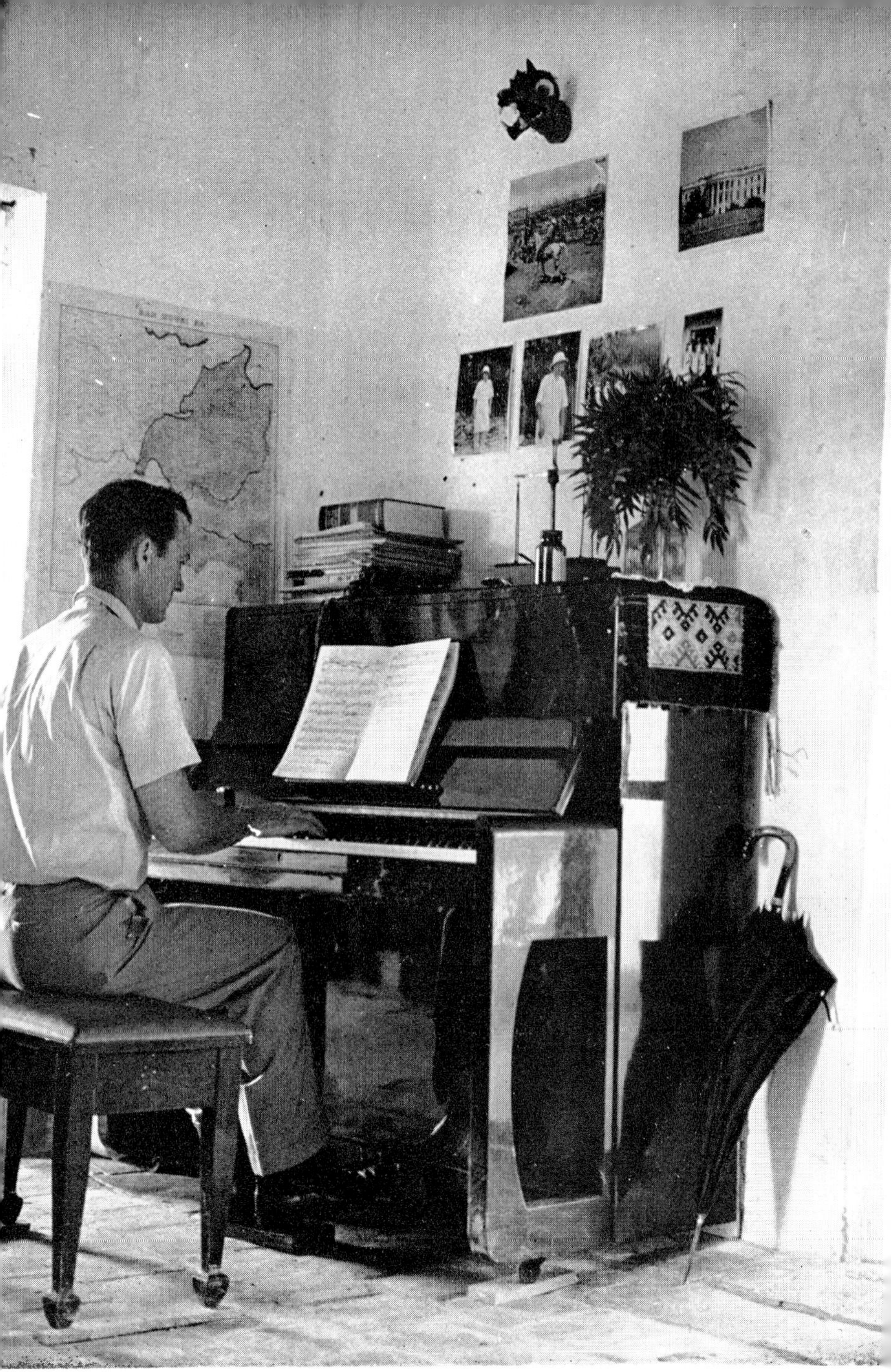

The zinc-lined piano, my pride and joy, gift of the Wilson Club of General Electric, Bridgeport, Conn.

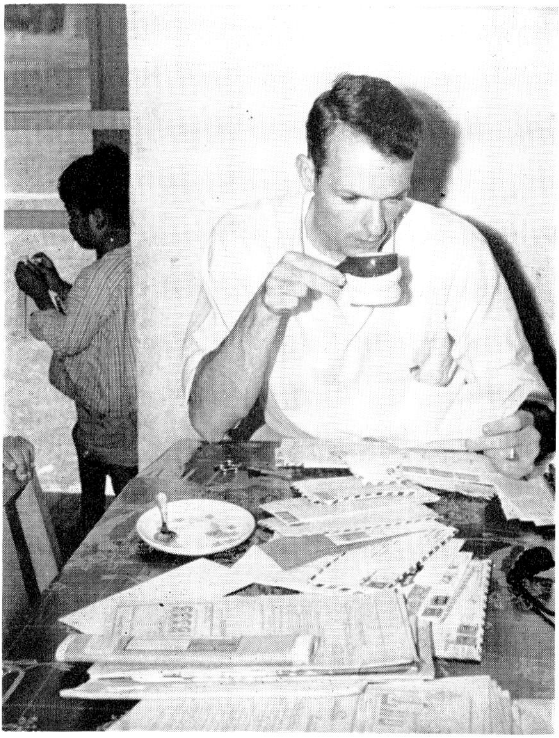

Mail call.

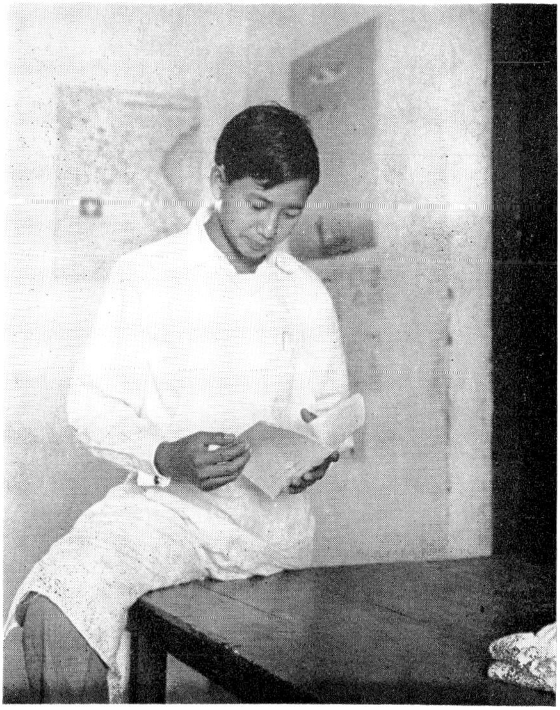

Studious Ngoan, a boy of the Black Thai tribe.

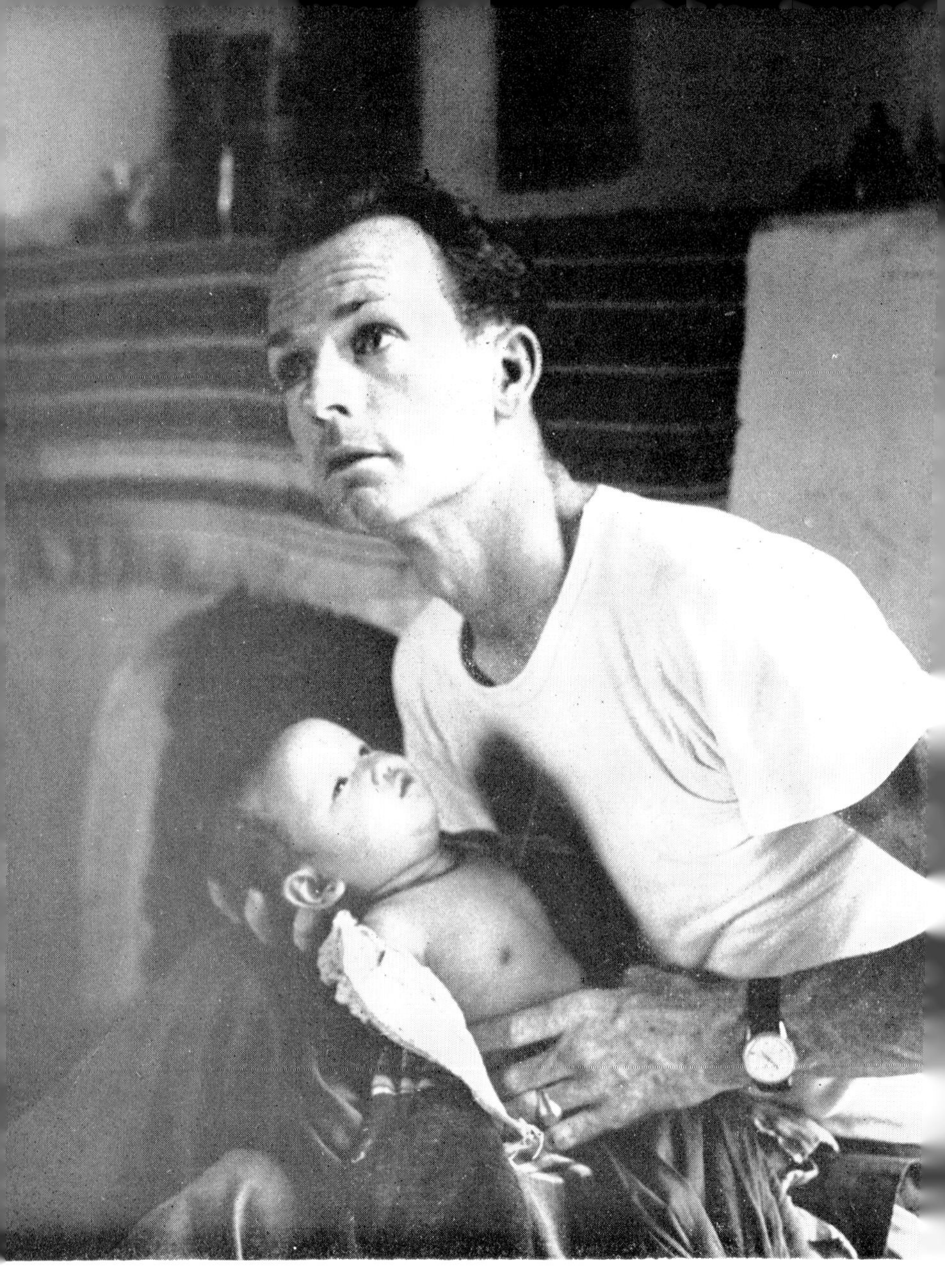

When a doctor feels helpless: a tiny life, which he knows will be brief.

A Kha Kho patient.

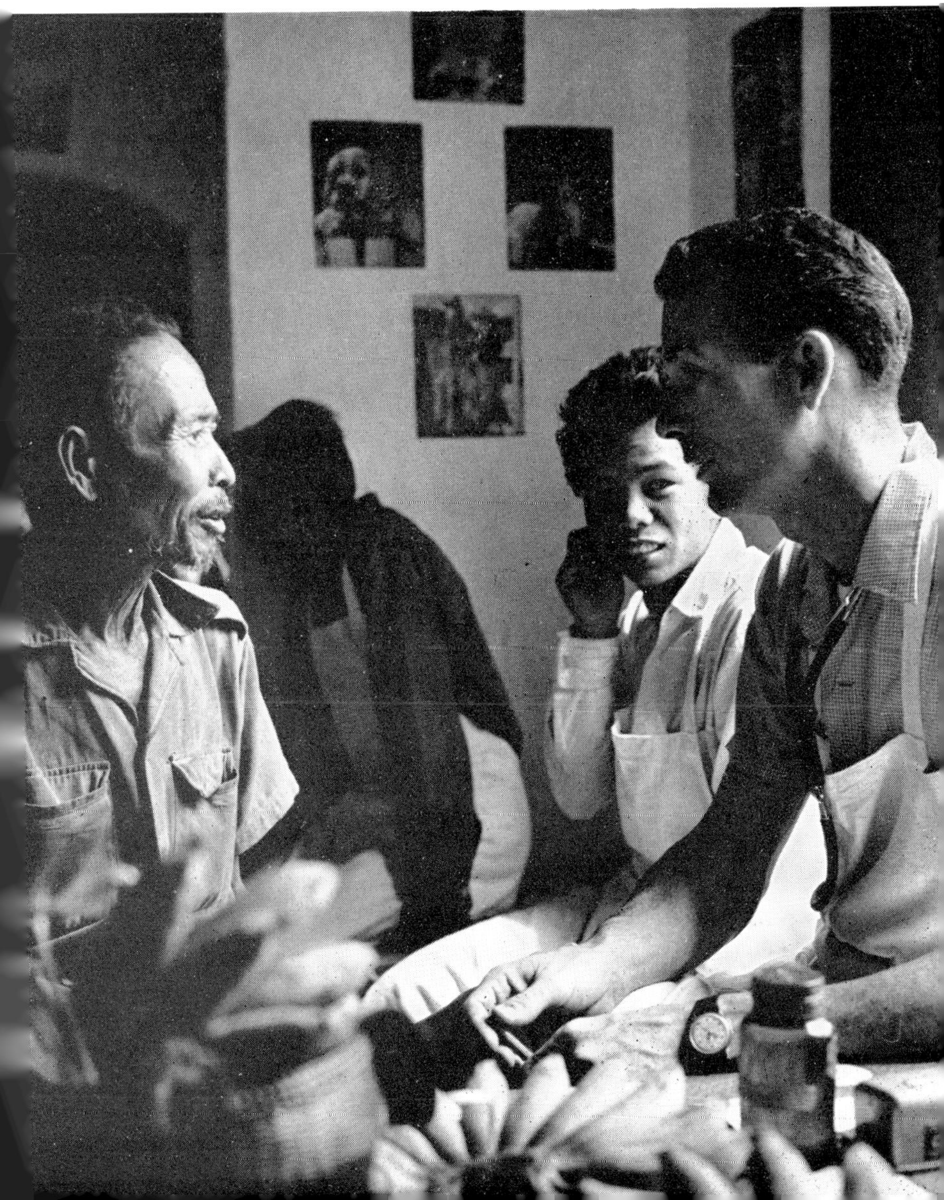

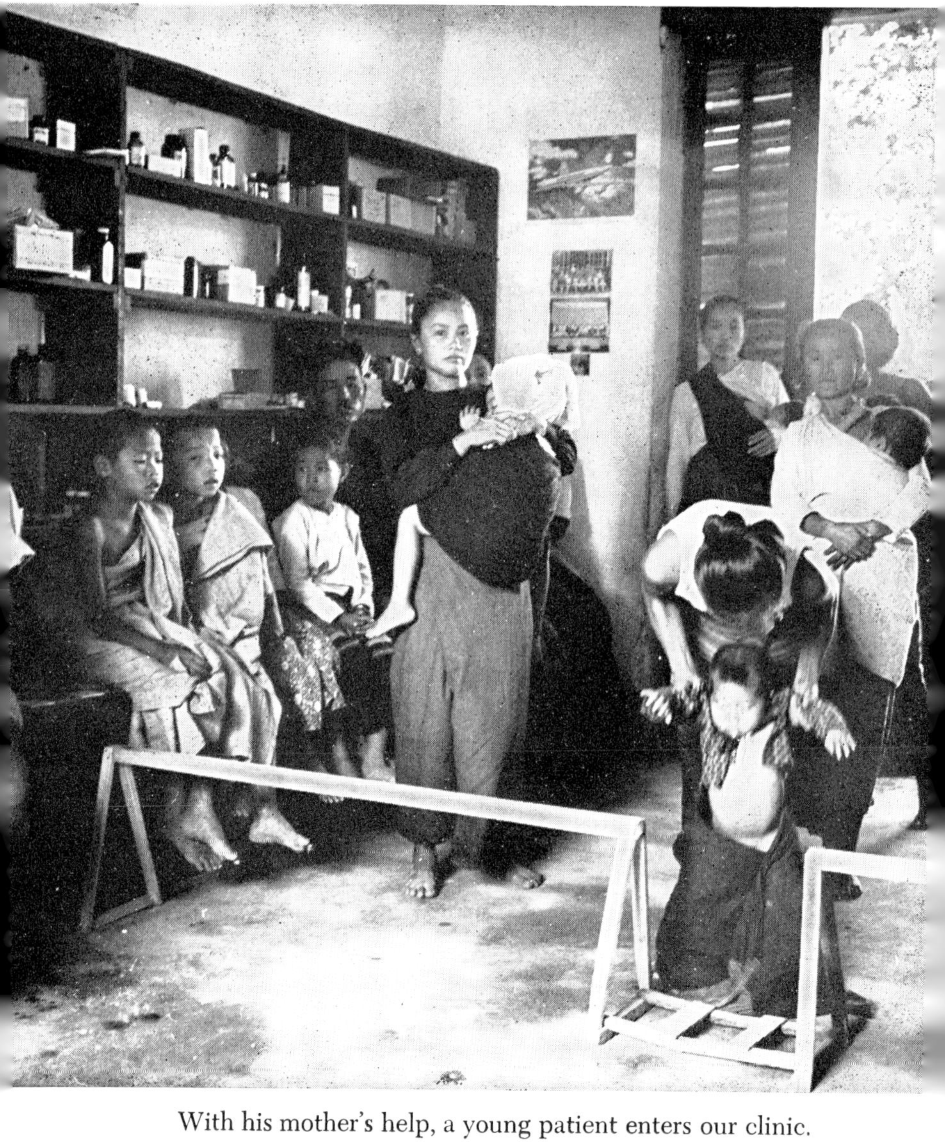

With his mother's help, a young patient enters our clinic.

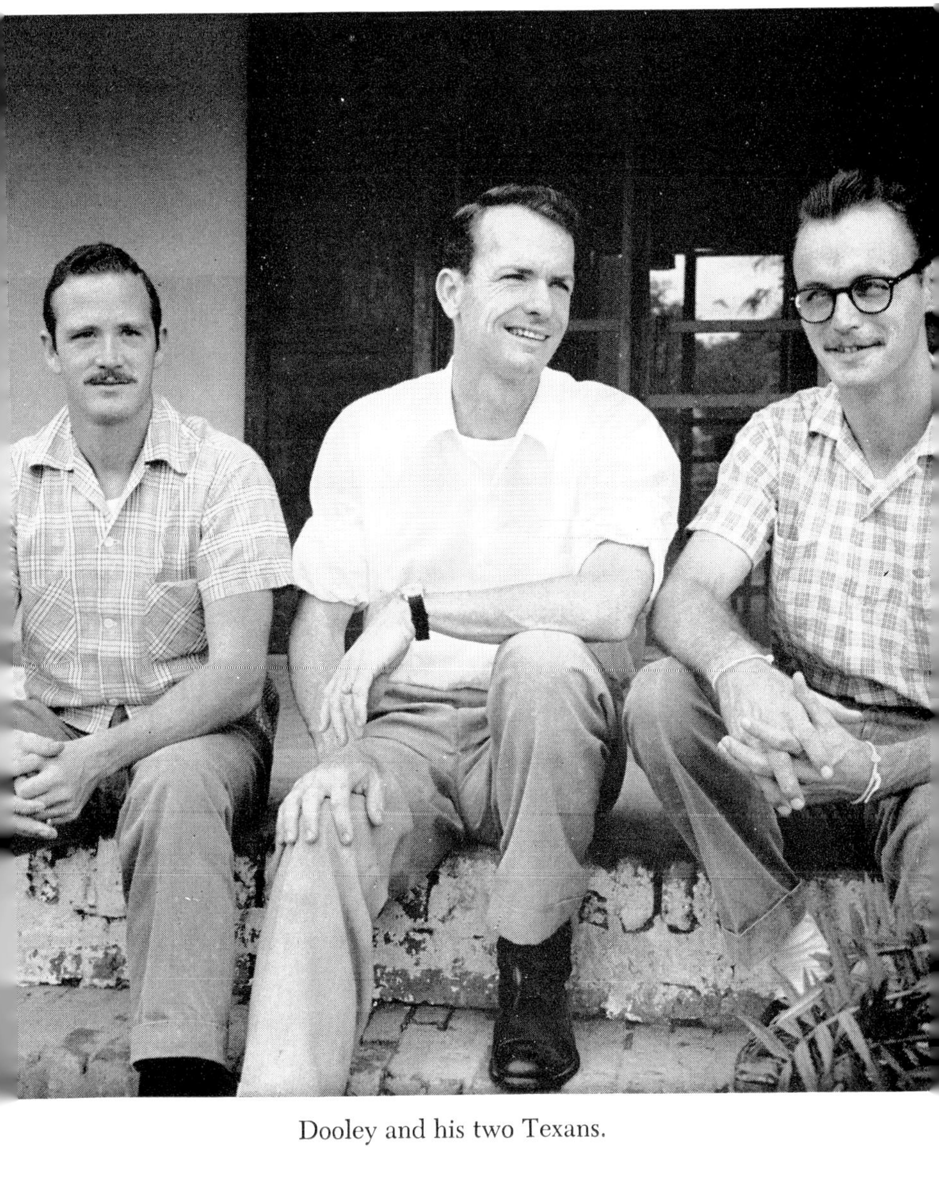

Dooley and his two Texans.

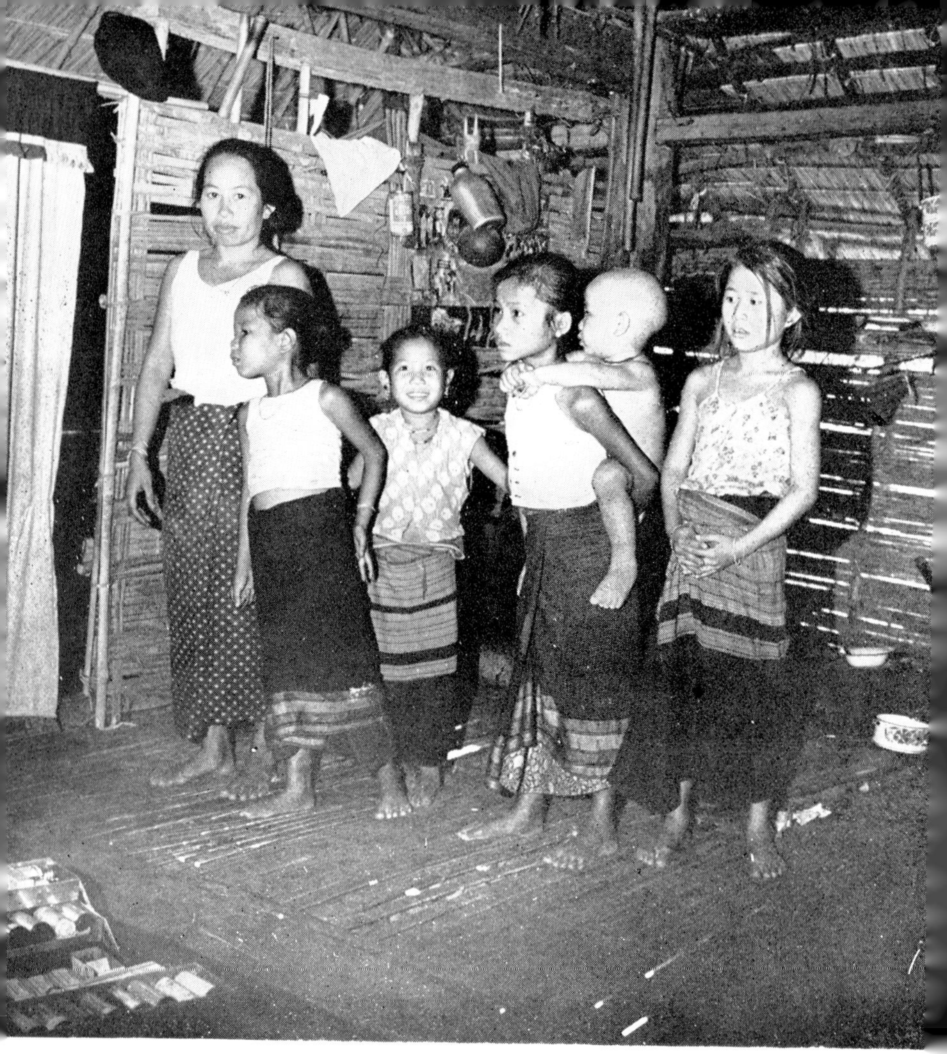

House call brings me inside a typical village dwelling. Note my medical bag on floor, lower left.

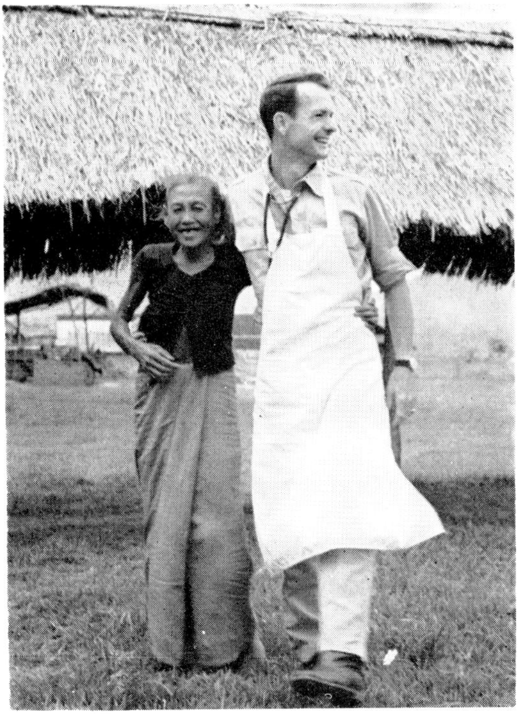

"Gravel Gertie," a witch doctor, with her admirer.

Main Street in Muong Sing.

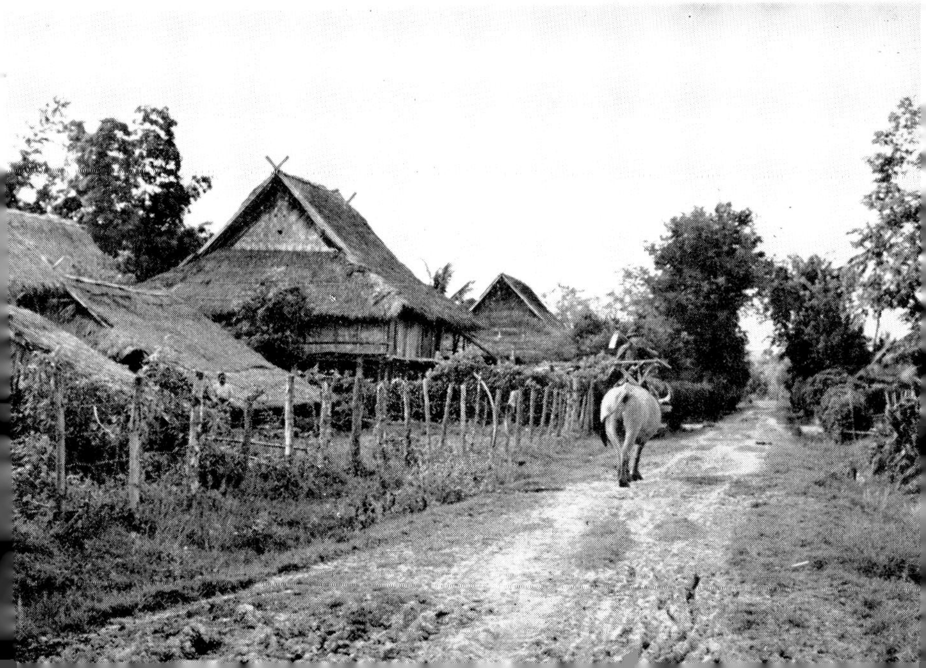

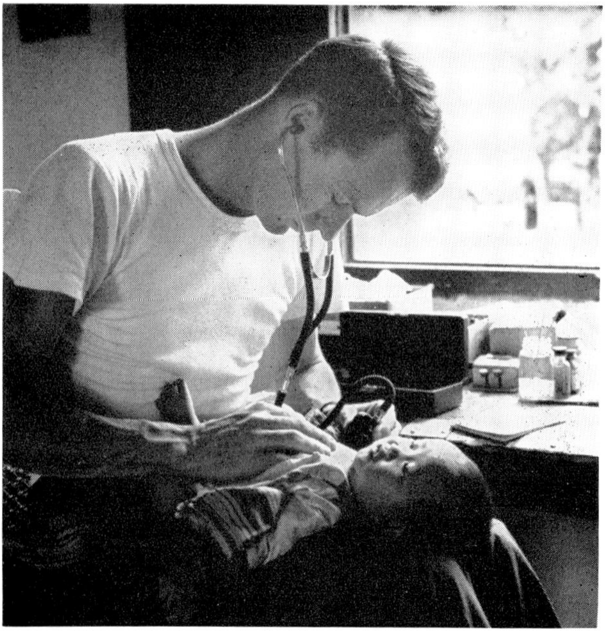

The heart-beat of Asia.

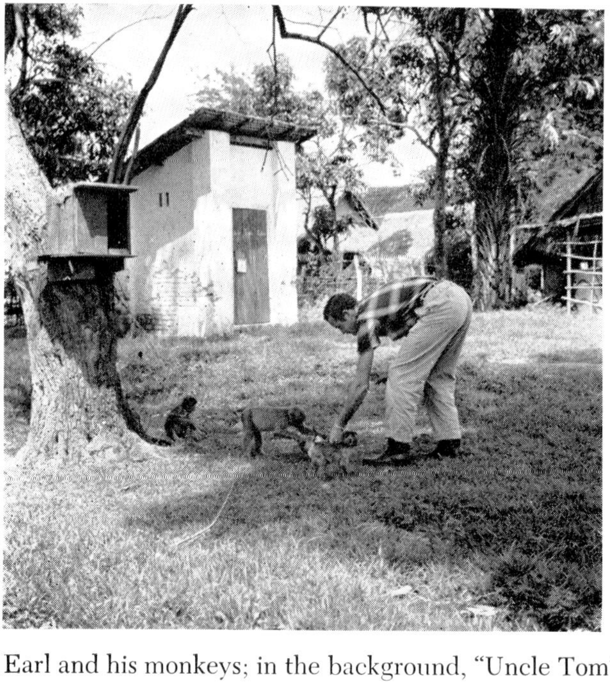

Earl and his monkeys; in the background, "Uncle Tom's Cabin."

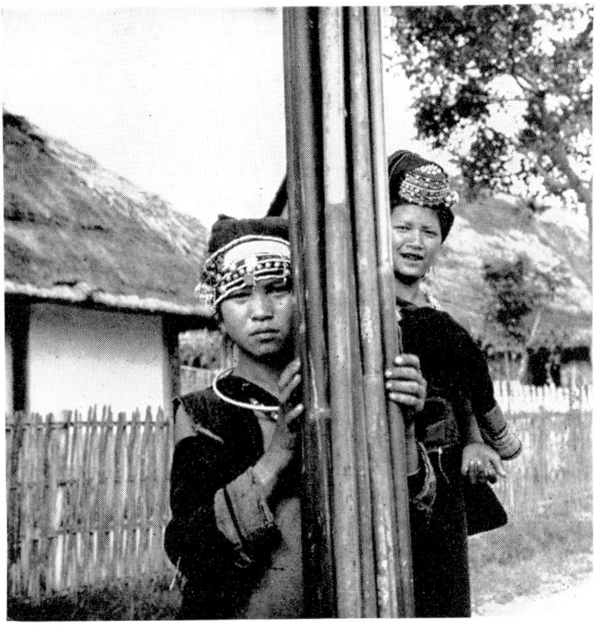

Two women of the Kha Kho tribe.

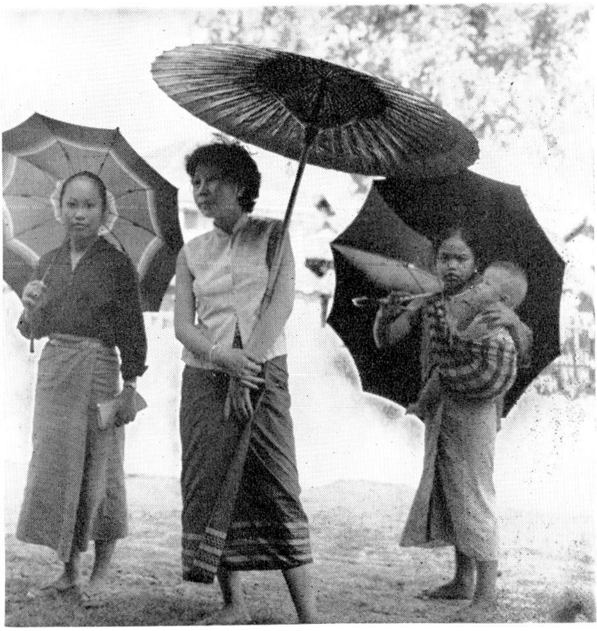

The Mayor's wife comes to visit.

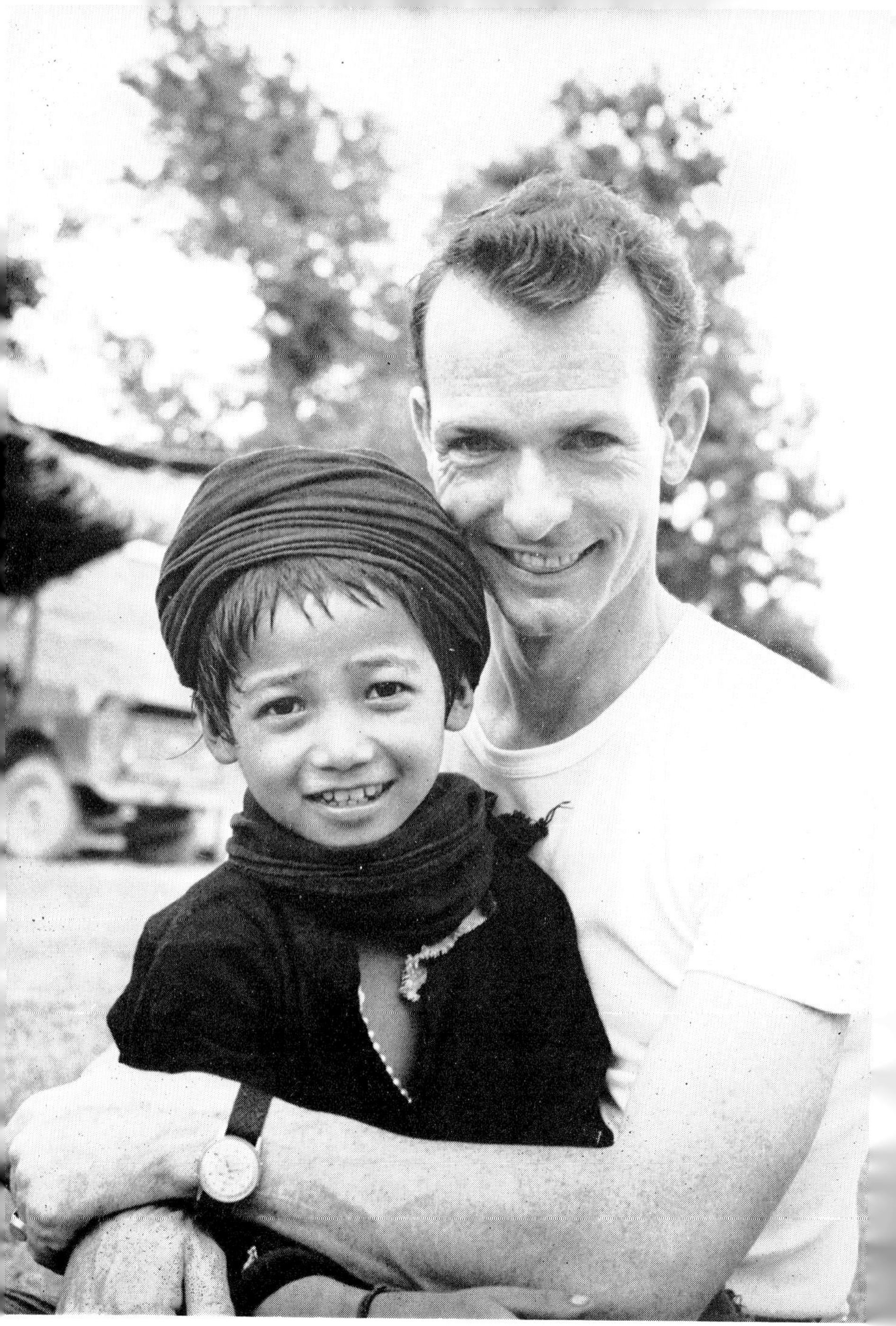

Tao Koo and his American friend.

SIX ·

"RESPECTFUL MEN OF MEDICINE"

Perhaps our hospital at Muong Sing was unattractive, whitewashed, utilitarian, and ugly. But it was also a compassionate candle in the darkness.

It only took a few weeks to put the clinic building in usuable shape. The clinic building, like our house, had three major rooms, plus two smaller ones on the side. One room was temporarily used as a ward. Later when the new ward building was finished, we made it over into an operating room. The room on the west side of the building was the dressing room and the small room behind it was the shot room. The large central room was the clinic.

The clinic was a long rectangular room, with the window at one end and the door at the other. Along each side the boys had built long high shelves. On the bottom of these shelves were five crates in which our gear had been shipped from America. These crates had been painted green and covered with linoleum. Everything in our hospital was painted green and covered with linoleum, a Dooley fixation.

We put up a foot-high railing across the center of the room. I sat in front of the window at the opposite end from the door. I had a desk on one side, the patient's chair in front of me, and interpreters on each side of me. Two students would stand against the shelves on my left. Two other students would stand in the shot room and watch from the adjoining door.

The sick man would come through an opening in the center railing, walk up to me and sit on the chair. With my interpreters and forty or fifty people behind the railing listening in, we would discuss this man's ailments. By having everyone listening in, many other people learned. "Oh, can you cure that kind of a thing, doctor?" they would ask. "My mother has the same problem." "Oh explain yourself better than that, Houmpenh," they would urge an old man. "Tell them what your problem is." It really added a touch of togetherness to our work, and after all there was a certain propaganda element in what we were doing.

After I discussed the problem with the patient and my students, the patient was sent to the shelves. There he would receive medicine from the students. I never gave any medicine to anyone. Nor did my two Americans. The Asian students would be told, "This man has pneumonia. Give him something for his pneumonia, some terramycin." The Asian student would then take the terramycin bottle from the shelf, put the correct number of capsules into an envelope, and give them to the patient. The Asian student would explain to the patient the dosage schedule, and would make such comments as "Why don't you wash your hands?" "Why didn't you bring your child back here last week?" "Why haven't you done what the doctor told you to do last week?"

This idea of Asians helping Asians is much superior to Americans helping Asians. When the patient received the medicine, he would turn to the Asian student and say, "*Cup Chai.*" They knew the help was American but they were grateful to the Asian student too. My Asian students will be here all their lives, I will not. I dispensed nothing, the Asians did.

The main theme of our work was to establish things so that Asians could maintain them. This included prestige, position, and pride.

If the patient had to have a shot, he was sent in through the door on my right, where we would tell the two students what to give—penicillin, streptomyocin, dramamine, and so on. A card was given to the patient with the number of shots that he would need. As the shot was given, the student would mark it off the card.

If the patient needed a dressing, he was sent to the dressing room which was the west end of the building. There on many low tables the patients would sit. Earl and Dwight would run this room much like a symphony conductor. With all the patients sitting, the Lao students would begin to treat the wounds, washing them, suturing them, cleaning them. Earl would say, "Wash that one with hydrogen peroxide." "Clean that one up with a little soap and water." "You had better take the stitches out of that one, they have been in long enough." "Better call Thanh Mo America in to look at this wound. It's kind of bad." By this system it was the Asians who cared for the wounds of the Asians and not the white men. To be sure, Earl and Dwight and I looked at many a wound and sutured hundreds of them. But as often as possible and to every extent possible the Asians took care of their own.

Earl and Dwight, though reluctant at first, later saw the wisdom of this action and carried it out even better than I. They taught the students how to suture by having them practice sewing their pants legs together. Many times a suture job would have to be done and I would merely tell Dwight to do it. Dwight in turn supervised Deng or some other student in doing the job. The Lao boys who did the suture job would take great pride in their work and give the patient their daily dressings with much compassion and interest.

The sick call started early in the morning, and ended up after high noon. The patients paid us in chickens, eggs and corn, and would say to our students, and to us, the most sublime utterance in any language—the words of gratitude. Two words, "Thank you."

The villagers who came to our clinic were wonderful people to see and know. Some were as frail as an El Greco saint. Others looked like mystic holy men, with wispy little beards of a hundred hairs. Others were fat and corpulent women who laughed and smiled, their bodies rippling with them. Many brought their spindly-legged, pot-bellied little children glumly perched on their hips, the pathos in the eyes of the mother almost matching the bleak look of death in the eyes of their children.

Many of the patients had beautiful Mongol features, delicate creamy skins and deep-set eyes. Others had bright almond eyes, or eyes so deep that one looked into bottomless pools. The children with bulging bellies and gaping wounds rapidly became healthy and husky. Several times the wretched sick came from huts where they lived on miserable straw pallets in dark rooms. They came to our bright clinic with colorful pictures on the walls and put themselves in the tender hands of my crew. And they were better even before they received their antibiotics. Some of the old men were like little walnuts, browned and wrinkled and withered. Sometimes straggling primitive hordes of human beings known as refugees would come. These silent people, witnesses to such horrors of Communism, are the sad song of humanity in our time.

Then there would be the bouncing healthy children who

would wait for sick call more interested in the show than in any particular illness. They would be energetically swishing, swatting, and thwacking, to keep the bugs away. The people at our clinic, in the high valley of Muong Sing, were just like the people who came to me in clinics in America. They had their share of meanness and magnificence. But there is something different about them because the prospect of curing sickness was a totally revolutionary concept to them. The villagers all their lives had thought it was impossible to be rid of malaria, goiter, rickets, dysentery and boils.

When we demonstrated to them that they need not have these things, it was an amazing and wonderful thing. The scarlet and black wounds that burst in their superb olive flesh were closed up with simple cleanliness. The dirty stumps of teeth were extracted with ease; no longer did they have a fetid or foul mouth. Soon the wretched patients with green-black sores, or inflamed bellies, would quietly become cured. They were the better for our having been there.

I also watched my American assistants at work. Earl Rhine's ease at handling people was beautiful to behold. He showered his time and attention on the wretched sick with a sad kind of joy. With grand aplomb he treated them all like visiting royalty. For example, one day a wizened old man came to him and gesticulated how he had an excruciating pain in his left knee. The old man explained very carefully that "the pain begins in my left knee and runs up the inside of my leg. The pain plunges into my pelvis, continues on up to my face and into my head." He went on to say that with some dizziness the pain would come out the tip of his nose and "then it falls to my knee, the other one." Earl listened very seriously and nodded his head with a solemn and professional mien that would have pleased the President of the American Medical Association. Then, with insight and knowledge, he said, "Oh, yes, of course. I completely understand. I suggest hot soaks for both knees."

Dwight Davis would jokingly call some haggard, snaggle-toothed old gal "honey," though this in no way ever indicated any superficiality of concern. Earl in turn examined each patient as though he were examining the king himself. Both men did a magnificent job. My patients risked too much compassion.

Each person was important as a person. I tried to get this view across to Earl and Dwight, only to find that they already fully realized its importance. Whether the child was a bleating mountain boy or the son of the local Mayor, he was important to Dwight and Earl because he was a child.

Earl had a love affair. Only Earl's "love" was a five-year-old girl whose slim little body had all the delicacy of the proverbial lotus flower. This midnight-eyed Asian girl would come to see Earl frequently. At the mature age of five she would blithely walk into our house and sit down, folding her hands gracefully in her lap as though they were simply two leaves that had fallen into her sarong. When she walked, she put each foot down as softly as trembling light. She never said one word to Earl during all the time that he knew her. And yet she came almost every day. From time to time Earl would be out on a river trip and she would come to the house, look around for Earl, and when she realized he was not there, she would go home. She had nothing to do with Dwight and me. She was Earl's love.

If Earl was there she would climb up on his lap, no matter what he was doing, and sit there in utter contentment until Earl was forced to put her down to do his work. She would then smile, clasp her hands in front of her face in the prayerful fashion of saying adieu, and "silently steal away."

It has been stated on high echelons in Washington that the success of American foreign policy in Asia depends primarily upon the image we create of America and Americans in the minds of Asian people. If this is true (and I believe it to be so), the image of Americans in the eyes of thousands of people in Muong Sing is the image of the gentility, compassion, and love of Dwight Davis and Earl Rhine.

Earl seemed more interested in dentistry than he did in medicine. His mossy-toothed dental patients swore by him. No matter what the dental problem might be, however, he had only one treatment, extraction. When I had to leave Laos on an emergency a year later, the first letter that I received from the boys included the statement that they had found a very small foot-powered dental drill and had purchased it—"hope you don't mind."

We all wore white coats in the clinic and Earl had one of the Lao student midwives embroider his name in Lao on his coat. The word Thanh Mo means "respectful man of medicine," though "Mo" also includes witch doctors. I am called Thanh Mo America. Earl was referred to as Thanh Mo Chep Keo which literally means "respectful man of medicine for pain in the teeth." This is the closest our village dialect comes to the word dentist.

Just before dawn, one of the first weeks we were in North Laos, we were torn from our sleep by the shrieks of a screaming woman. She was only a few feet from our window. I lunged to the window and saw several men huddled over something. The moonlight was bright. I jumped out of the window to the ground a few feet below, yelling for Earl and Dwight. They leaped after me and immediately the clump of men raced away. They left a sagging limp figure on the ground. I bent down and recognized the bloody mass of a young woman we had recently hired. She was working for us as payment for the delivery of her child. She had no home, her husband was in the army, and she had come quite some distance to our new American hospital for her delivery. We had hired her to give her a place to eat and live for a few months.

Even by moonlight I could tell she had been brutually stabbed with long dagger-like knives. Dozens of deep wounds pumped blood from her body. The bundle on the ground by her side was her newborn baby. He had also been stabbed. The men that we saw running away were the ones who had attacked them. Why?

We carried her bleeding body into the hospital a few feet away, and tried to get her blood-soaked clothes off. Intravenous fluid was started immediately and we began to try to stop the bleeding from all of the stab wounds around her body. It was futile. Within a few minutes she stopped breathing entirely. She had lost too much blood. The floor underneath the operating room table was wet with congealed blood. We baptized her and turned our attention to the baby.

Meanwhile, quite a large crowd had gathered, including the Chief of the Military Battalion and the Chief of Police. Chai, Earl, Dwight and I were operating on the baby to sew up the multiple deep lacerations, which tore through the muscles and down to the bone of both the arm and leg. We repaired the infant, and gave him to a nurse who took the child from the awesome scene. Then we went to the house and collapsed from the shock of it all. Everything seemed so useless. Why would anyone attack this young woman? What ever prompted such a hideous atrocity so close to our house? Was this an indication of hatred for us?

We carefully wrapped the dead girl's body, and she was buried the next morning. Her child was adopted by some people in the neighborhood. For many weeks everyone was speaking about the murder—and there were many reasons given for it. The one that seemed to be generally adopted was that she was having a love affair with a soldier and the soldier killed her.

This seemed hard to understand, as she had just given birth to a child a few days beforehand. Also the Chief of the Military claimed that he had caught the soldier and put him in prison, though no one else ever saw him. This included our Lao military students who lived in the fortress just a few feet from this prison cell. It is my personal belief that this was a Communist maneuver in order to frighten us out of North Laos. It frightened us indeed, but not out of North Laos.

What it did do was bring several things sharply and clearly into focus for all three of us. It was not a new experience for me; I have seen the anguish of atrocity. All my years of training, of study and experience were focused that night on that mutilated young girl before me. Yet at dawn the girl was devoid of breath and blood and life itself—dead. The horror of this night was simply an introduction for Dwight and Earl to what they would have to bear for the many months ahead.

From the date of our arrival we were constantly in the processes of building. As soon as we got the house in order and the clinic finished, we started to work building the new ward. Behind the clinic building some 50 yards was a small shell [illegible] old building. Attached to this building on three sides were a series of grass huts, occupied by the wives of some of the military. We gently, yet firmly, had these ladies evicted and we took over this area for our ward. The huts were torn off, a wall or two was knocked down, another built up, much cementing, scrubbing and painting and we soon had for ourselves a three-roomed ward. The ward had mat space for twenty or twenty-five and I suppose in an emergency we could jam in a few more. We covered all the holes and spots that would not take paint with pictures and postcards sent to us from people all over the world.

We also found that our patients, of their own free will, painted some of our walls. They painted them with signs and symbols of witchcraft and black magic. The tribal people of North Laos wallow in superstition, black magic, necromancy and sorcery. There are as many legends as there are mountain peaks. There are as many herbs as there are trees. Our working in this area demanded a constant awareness of the power of witchcraft and black magic. So our walls even displayed our peaceful coexistence with witchcraft.

The army sent over to us daily working parties to help build. The whole compound was leveled off. What had been a patchwork of sinkholes, buffalo wallows, ditches and hillocks became a level, clean hospital compound. We even transplanted grass. Around the hospital compound (about the size of a football field) we had a ditch dug and a barbed wire fence erected. The ditch was to keep out water and the fence to keep out buffaloes; both had a tendency to collect on our compound. Earl, with all of the knowledge of a Midwestern farmer, planted a vegetable garden. The tomatoes grew to be succulent and large, but we rarely got a chance to eat them. The jungle monkeys got there first. Si planted flower gardens all around the hospital and they grew in profusion. We soon had a lovely looking hospital compound, primitive, utilitarian, but neat, clean, and whitewashed.

As far as witch doctors are concerned, they have several techniques. One of the types of magic that they use is a defensive thing. They have fetishes and objects that are endowed with certain magical powers. I have a gift given me by people of a mountain village. It is a stone with a Buddha carved on it. The stone is wrapped in a tiny net of silver. This will protect me against two things, bullets and black magic. The people believe these chains around their necks and little bags with pieces of silver are extremely powerful, not unlike certain talismans used in Africa. However, when I was at medical school I saw many a patient wearing a copper penny on a chain around his neck. And as a matter of fact, I know one very sophisticated woman in the American community in Laos who wears copper bracelets to keep arthritis away. (Perhaps we really shouldn't attack witchcraft too vehemently.)

When the witch doctor talks to patients, he really elicits something like a clinical history. He asks the patient what he is wearing and how long he's been wearing it. He asks if the patient has any talismans or amulets around. He asks what was the position of the moon when the sickness began. What dreams had he been having? The witch doctor then sits down to read long passages from folded "bibles."

One afternoon Chai's wife was quite sick and he called me over to her house. I found one of the old gentlemen of the village, a sorcerer, sitting cross-legged with a long fanfold of something like cardboard. He was reading ancient Pali script. On the floor before him Chai was sitting in a white surgical gown from my modern hospital, listening and offering worship to witchcraft. If you can't fight 'em, join 'em.

Often the witch doctor would tie black and white strings around the affected part, or rub ashes on the forehead, or lay leaves under the ground around the sick patient. They also fill a small bowl with eggs and rice and a small candle. In some areas I have seen them make little mud images of horses and cows and elephants and lay these on the bowl of rice as offerings to the evil spirits.

When I had a visiting surgeon with me one time, we went to see a child who was lying on a bank of leaves. Herbs are of importance to these people. The villagers believe that illness is due to the presence of an evil spirit and that lying on these herbs would chase the spirit away.

I found that the primitive people of our high valley were very anxious to be cut open. They have no fear of my scalpel and seem to think that I can actually cut the evil spirit out. One man of the Kha Kho tribe was delighted to have me operate on his wife because he knew that I would have to turn on the light in the operating room. He seemed to think that to chase the evil spirit, all I had to do was make a cut, let the light shine in, and the evil spirit would flee. I wish it were that simple.

The Kha Kho tribe, of the high hills, paint their teeth black. We spoke to one of our friends of this tribe asking about the black teeth. He summed the whole thing up in words that I had heard many years previously in North Viet Nam: "Who would want white teeth like a dog?" The men paint their teeth black when they begin to get interested in girls. The girls paint their teeth at puberty. This ceremony takes place with a celebration. The substance with which they paint their teeth stays on for a lifetime. They take the bark of a certain tree and cook it down until it becomes a thick paste. This is mixed with other ingredients and then is rubbed on the teeth every day for seven days.

The only time they reapply this is when they become very sick. They believe that by reapplying it, they will have better health. Many times I have seen patients sitting in my ward, blackening their teeth again.

There are many different tribes in the area. The Kha Kho are the most primitive, and the Thai Lu the most predominant. The Thai Lu, who have a more developed civilization than the Kha Kho, stand tall and straight. They are angular and thin, and though they have Mongoloid features they are not as squat as the hill people. The Thai Lu tattoo their bodies, the men from the knees to the waistline, covering practically every inch of that area, and the women tattoo small figures on their arms and words across their backs. All this is supposed to give them "strength," and protect them by inserting good spirits under their skins.

In all of Indo-China this custom of tattooing goes back to prehistoric times. There is an ancient legend which says that a mythical king ordered the fishermen of all his realm to tattoo the monsters of the sea on their arms. This, it was believed, would protect them against crocodiles. In the ancient court of Annam, in central Viet Nam, the kings tattooed images of dragons on themselves. The dragon is not only the symbol of Viet Nam but of all Indo-China. You often see dragons undulating across the roofs of pagodas, tattooed on people's skins, painted on walls, carved in homes. The dragon is one of the four symbolic animals engraved in Buddhism, the others being the unicorn, the phoenix, and the turtle.

Although I have never run across a dragon personally, many people have described them to me. Chai claims he has seen many. They tell me that the dragon has a head which is shaped like a deer's, with great horns, and his monster eyes stick way out of their sockets. The dragons of North Laos, I was told, have the ears of a water buffalo and the long body and tail of a reptile. Chai says they have scales like fish, but where the fins should be there are large claws, like a vulture's.

The dragon is a very marvelous creature. "He's even more marvelous than Americans," Chai says. The top of the dragon's head always has a decorative area which is supposed to be the mark of intelligence. The dragon can live either underground, in the water, or in the air. He can swim, walk or fly. And the dragon spits a certain kind of vapor which he can transform into fire or water at will. Of course everybody knows that dragons are immortal. The people of North Laos reconfirm this frequently. There is one dragon in the area who is supposed to have lived down our road for 5,000 years. In spite of these terrible characteristics, the dragon is not considered an evil thing. On the contrary, the dragon has always been a symbol of nobility and power in China, and some of this dragon culture has sifted down to North Laos too.

In view of their more positive qualities of durability, intelligence and power, I sometimes think I would like to have an official dragon attached to each of the MEDICO teams around the world. How about it, Dr. Comanduras?

SEVEN ·

TAKE A WALK WITH ME

Our ward is something unique to see. We have three rooms which we majestically called "Ward A," "Ward B," and "Ward C." Each room is small, about eighteen feet in width and just about the length of two average American beds. As you enter the door there is a bed to the left and another to the right. At the other end of the room is one large platform. We lay bamboo mats on the platforms and hang individual mosquito nets; in this way a platform can sleep five or six.

On a typical day of making rounds, you would find a small girl of the Kha Mou tribe on Mat 1 in Ward A. She is a little reluctant to talk to you, but her father and mother who are staying here with her are not. The mother herself had a large tumor which we removed surgically. While she was here we realized that her child was wracked with pneumonia. We are treating both of them.

On Mat 4, we have an old Yao man who lives high in the mountains in a village called Ban Chao Mai. He had had a bladder stone almost all of his life, but the old goat was sort of indestructible. We had a lot of trouble with him before surgery, but finally we removed a stone just a little smaller than a tennis ball. Yes, a tennis ball. I cannot speak his dialect, but Chai can. The old man said: "Doctor America, you can have my bladder stone. I don't want it." It was obvious, however, that this old gent was doing fine—not complaining for a change and, by all signs and symptoms, much improved. We call him "Old Indestructible" because he has had such a difficult time post-surgically.

Over on the other part of the platform we have another Yao, a small boy nearly blind in both eyes. He has an entropion, a disease that is caused from the scarring of the lower or upper eyelid. The inside of the eyelid scars from many repeated or from constant infections. The scar makes the eyelids turn in. The eyelashes therefore constantly rubbing on the eyeball causing more irritation to the eye. This in turn causes more scar, more contraction and more inturning of the lash on the eyeball. The surgical correction is merely to excise an eliptical piece of skin off of the top of the eyelid, leaving a gap in the skin. The lower portion of this area is then pulled up over the denuded area to the top part of the eliptical excised area. The eyelid is made narrow and in pulling the skin up it turns the eyelid up, too. The eyelashes no longer rub on the eyeball. If surgery is not done, the repeated infections will cause the boy to be totally blind by the time he is ten. After surgery he looks a great deal better. With cortisone drops in the eyes, the corneal irritation diminishes rapidly and vision returns. Now he will see as well as any child.

A third patient on the platform is a lady getting over a blazing attack of malaria. As is so often the case, these people exist on the brink of malnutrition. One or two days of high fever will push them off this ledge and they fall into a negative balance. Their ankles and bellies bloat up, they become extremely sick and emaciated in a staggeringly short time. This woman's malaria was cured with Camesquin, about eighty cents worth in a day. Now she is on protein extracts like Sustagen and the Meals for Millions. Her condition is mightily improved and after a few more days of convalescence she can go home.

Walk out on the porch now to the next door, into Ward B. Here we have a small boy whose name is Guntar. He is on Mat 1 on the left. Guntar belongs to the Kha Kho tribe. He claims to be seven years old. By the Buddhist calendar this may be true. By our calendar he is closer to six. A few weeks ago his father shot a tiger with an old flintlock. In wild exuberance the lad ran up to the body of the tiger. The animal, not yet dead, lunged at the child mauling him terribly. The boy's whole leg was practically torn off and blood loss and shock brought him close to death. By the time they got him to us his leg was just a bloated glob of infected flesh and pus. We feared it would be necessary to amputate at the thigh to prevent the poison of that nearly gangrenous limb from permeating his frail body. But we tried antibiotics on him first. The lad is doing very well now, after many days of hot soaks, terramycin, and good old-fashioned TLC ("tender loving care").

Frequently at night we show a movie on the wall of our house. Some 1,000 people sit on the grass and watch in wonder. Little Guntar loves the movies. I think movies have just as much therapeutic value as antibiotics. Walt Disney gave me a 16 mm. version of *Dumbo*. *Dumbo* has enchanted North Laos, and the children watch for him every time we show this movie. They never seem to tire of it. "What a wonderful land America must be," they say. "They have huge elephants and the elephants are pink and green and blue and purple. And some of these elephants have ears so big that they can fly through the air." *Dumbo* is winning friends in the ten-year-old bracket for sure.

The other patients in this ward are a sad assortment of malaria, dysentery, skin disease, malnutrition, and other maladies of filth, ignorance, and privation.

In Ward C we have a Meo woman and her husband. The Meo woman has a tumor in the abdomen which we are going to remove very soon. She is too anemic and too loaded with intestinal worms now. After these are cleaned out and her blood iron brought closer to normal, we will operate.

There are also some Kha Kho tribesmen in Ward C. One of them is a leper. There is not much we can do for him except keep him clean. Leprosy is not very contagious, contrary to Biblical beliefs.

We have several tuberculars in this ward, one of them a thirty-five-year-old man, who belongs to the Thai Dam tribe. We also have in this ward a very attractive young woman who came to us from the village near Nam Tha. Her husband is a member of the police force and he was able to get her on a special plane to be sent to us. She has tuberculosis and other diseases of malnutrition. However, she is doing very well now; her eyes are brightening up and she is a very lovable person. All of the police officers in town here (eight of them) come over every day to visit and bring her food. They take very good care of her. The deep sense of family among these Asians is a wonderful thing to behold.

Now I can hear someone saying, "My gosh, keeping children in the same room with tuberculars." Yes, it's bad, but there is such a tremendous amount of tuberculosis here. We gave our cases streptomycin for fourteen days, and built up their cachetic bodies with Deca Vi Sol and Sustagen. Though not cured, they are always discharged improved, with instructions in diet and some explanation of the principles of contagion.

I do not want to enlarge upon the incidence of tuberculosis in Laos, because to be scientifically correct I would have to have laboratory smears and x-rays, but I would estimate that one in ten over the age of forty has tuberculosis; and one in five over the age of fifty. We do not use any new drugs and we do not devote a great deal of time to the treatment of tuberculosis because I am more interested in cases which can be readily cured rather than the chronic cases that require long-term treatment. Our emphasis is on the more readily treatable diseases.

In Ward C we have a lady with a bad dental infection. The whole side of her left cheek is missing and there is a gaping hole. She can stick her tongue out the side of her face where her cheek should be. There is just one thin bridge of tissue on the side of the mouth running from the upper lip to the lower lip. We tried plastic surgery on her, but it was unsuccessful. We will wait now until a visiting plastic surgeon comes and we can do a more complicated skin graft.

Ward rounds are held by Dwight and Earl every morning just a little after dawn. I make rounds in the afternoon, seeing only the cases Earl and Dwight feel I must see. These two American boys are really tops. It is a wondrous thing to watch them care for the wretched. They use so well the hot towels of caution and the aspirin of compassion. They soothe the small child and they help and quiet and give strength to the old. My men have high courage, goodness, patience, and constancy. Our small ward is a veritable chapel of compassion.

My interpreter Chai has been with me since I first came to Asia in 1956. In *The Edge of Tomorrow* I told how I met him, and how he refused to swim in the Nam Lick river because he hadn't been checked out with the spirits. Chai is a very competent Asian corpsman, yet he still reverts back to his black magic when he feels that my terramycin and surgery are not quite adequate. After he recovered from his first month having yellow jaundice, he pitched in with the enthusiasm which so endeared him to us.

Neither Earl nor Dwight speak French, though Dwight does understand some due to his ability in Spanish. As soon as we arrived in Laos I knew I would have to find an English-speaking interpreter. They used to be difficult to find, but since American influence in Laos is increasing and all Asians want to learn English, the situation is improving. A friend in the American Economic Mission runs an English language school. This is not under any formal program, but just his own personal contribution to the people of Asia. I asked him if he would find someone in his school who could work for us, and he said he would.

The next night he brought to the home of Hank Miller a short, slightly stooped young boy, who didn't look a day over fourteen, as a candidate to be my interpreter. I was a little aghast to think that my conversations with certain of the tougher tribes would have to be handled through this little boy. I spoke to him in English and though he did have some competence, he was reluctant, fearful and overly polite. At first I thought that this lad would never work. On the other hand I realized how frightened he must be, how anxious he was for the job, and his youth perhaps would make him malleable. I put him on the next plane to the north and told him he would be interpreter for Earl and Dwight. His name was Ngoan.

It took no time at all for Ngoan to become a very intimate part of the team, and to become as beloved as a brother. Chai would interpret for me and Ngoan would interpret for Earl and Dwight. Chai has always been my shadow, Ngoan is now shadow for Earl and Dwight. We kidded him so much about being stoop-shouldered that he soon learned to stand up straight. Eating the kind of food that we ate, he soon filled out and became a healthier and stronger boy. He was constantly studying. Every free moment that he had he was studying one of his books.

Later we had correspondence courses in simple language sent from America on which he worked diligently. Every time someone would say a word that he did not understand, he would write it in his little notebook and look it up later. Although his translations were a bit stiff, nevertheless they were accurate. The great strides that this boy made in the fifteen months he was with us was impressive.

One day we went up to the China frontier to see if any refugees were escaping, and to take a general look around it. We drove to a village a few miles from ours, climbed out of the jeep and began to hike. We had some of our soldier students with us as well as Si, Owi, and La. Just for comfort we brought along a map that showed the cartographic presence of the Communistic frontier. In these heavy hills and jungles I am always afraid of stepping three feet too far and ending up in China.

It was a beautiful day, the sun high, the sky blue, and there was a certain feeling of abandonment. This break from the dull monotony of misery was a good thing. As we walked in the high rain forest, Ngoan told us this story:

"The village where I was born looks like this valley. I was born in a village called Song La which is not very far from Dien Bien Phu. I, of the tribe of the Black Thai Dam, do not really live in Viet Nam or in Laos. Our tribe lives all across this land. This land belonged to our tribe long before France divided it up and called one part Vietnam and one part Laos.

"My country is very beautiful, but I do not ever remember anything but the blood of war in my days. In 1946 war was tearing the flesh of the valley of Song La. When the war destroyed my own village, my family was scattered. Some were taken prisoners, some of us escaped, and I got a job with a French soldier. I did his laundry. The soldier was very good to me. I was only eight or nine or ten, depending upon how you count. When this soldier was transferred to Dien Bien Phu, he took me with him. I then went to Hanoi, the great capital of North Viet Nam. I was his coolie. When 1954 came the fortress of Dien Bien Phu fell to the Communists, and I am told they had some big treaty somewhere and that the war was over."

(I thought to myself as Ngoan spoke that I, too, remember the fall of the fortress of Dien Bien Phu and for good reason. In 1954 this fortress was conquered by the Communists, just after June's Geneva Treaty. At that moment I was a Navy doctor running the refugee camp, not more than sixty kilometers from where Ngoan was living in North Viet Nam.)

"When I was in Hanoi," Ngoan continued, "I heard of the people leaving the north because they did not want to live under Communism. I did not want to live under the Communists because I had seen what their war had done, and I decided that I would leave too. I asked the soldier if he would take me, but he said that he could not. He said that he was very sorry but that they were unable to take their coolies with them." (However, the French did make a request to the American representatives in Saigon, and one day early in 1955, a few months before the Communists took over Hanoi, a group of American airplanes came to Hanoi.)

"All of the tribe of the Black Thai who were scattered in the mountains and in the city of Hanoi got together, because we were told that American airplanes would fly us to a free land very near by. We all climbed on airplanes which scared me and amazed me very much. I found my brother at the airport. He, too, was waiting for escape. I had not seen him for many years. The American airplanes were large and terribly frightening. They flew us to a village called Xieng Khouang in North Laos." Xieng Khouang is about a hundred miles straight west of the Vietnamese Black Thai tribal area of Song La. The area of Xieng Khouang is a tribal area of the Thai Dam also, though geographically it is in Laos. The Communists had not taken over this part of Indo-China. Here the Thai Dam could live in peace.

We sat by a mountain stream, as Ngoan continued: "I lived in Xieng Khouang for another year. Now that I was a man of thirteen or fourteen years old, I had to do gardening and farming work. I never owned any land, so I always had to work for other people and I did not like this. When I heard from my friends that the Lao government was going to resettle the Black Thai refugees further away from the Vietnam border, I decided to go too.

"I was then herded on more airplanes and flown down to the capital of Laos, Vientiane. In Vientiane I got a job as a waiter in a restaurant. When my brother came he got a job working in the garage for the United States Overseas Mission people. While he was there he met a Doctor Taeed, who was a member of the Bahai faith. Doctor Taeed was very good to my brother, and my brother told Doctor Taeed about me.

"A few days later Doctor Taeed took me to his small clinic. You know, Dr. Taeed takes care of the Americans in U.S.O.M., so I worked in his clinic as the clean-up boy. He also let me go to his school to begin to study English.

I was very pleased and proud to have an opportunity to study English. Dr. Taeed is a good man. He has done a great deal for my tribe, Black Thai. Everybody else says that we are no good, that we are only a tribe to be servants, to be slaves. I do not think this is true."

Earl, Dwight and I listened to Ngoan intently. We were enchanted by the way he spoke, by the clarity of his statements, the poignancy and tragedy that had been his very young life. Today he is only eighteen years old and yet he has seen more unhappiness and tragedy than most people who live to be eighty.

I said to him, "Well, Ngoan, how did you ever get to me?" Ngoan said, "I worked for Dr. Taeed for a period of eight months. I worked very hard to learn to speak English and then one day Dr. Taeed came to me and said, 'Ngoan, would you like to have a job with Dr. Dooley, the Thanh Mo America?' But I did not know what the word 'job' meant. When he explained it to me, I was frightened because I did not think my English was strong enough to be an interpreter for a doctor. But I did want to have the chance, and so he took me to the house of Mr. Miller to meet you. And now I am with you and I am very happy."

We frequently heard what life was like on the other side of the Bamboo Curtain, the curtain of terror. The most vivid example came one afternoon when Earl, Dwight and I were building a small cage. We had been given a tiny Himalaya sun-bear as a gift. We were building a cage which was only a few feet high and a few feet wide. This cage was going to be put up in a tree at the back of the house, and the little bear would be kept in it.

While we were building the cage, a man came and squatted on his haunches and watched us. He kept watching us. Finally he began to cry. I called for my Yunnanese interpreter who came and spoke to the man. Soon the interpreter began to cry. The man had told him this story:

"I live in the large village on the other side of that mountain slope. The Communists came to our village several months ago to build a commune. You know the communes of China, doctor. The Communists come into a village of some 600 huts and they destroy 50 huts in the middle of the village. And all the men are put into the huts on the south side and all the woman into the huts on the north side. The children are taken away to live in another village. The old folks are taken to the village with the children. The Communists thus break up the family.

"All the cooking utensils are smelted down into one general cooking area. All the harvested rice must be put into the village commune. There is no tax, all the rice goes into the same basket."

The man continued to cry, sobbing more strongly than before. Earl, Dwight and I sat down on a log and listened to him more intently. He continued: "My wife had beriberi because she did not eat enough rice. One day my son and I were harvesting our rice, and my son put two handfuls of harvested rice into his pocket instead of putting it into the village commune. He was caught as he returned to the village.

"He had committed a crime against the state, as all food belongs to the state. This was the highest crime he could be accused of. The rice had not even been decorticated, it was just the raw rice. Because he had committed a crime against the state, the state punished him. The chief of the commune built a small cage just about the size of this cage that you are building for your bear. My son was put into the cage. It was so small that he could not stand nor sit, but had to bend over with his head jammed down hard and one leg thrust out through the bars on the side of the cage. The cage was put into the middle of the village square. Around it was put a roll of barbed wire, and around that the guards.

"Under the direct sun my son stood in this cage, having all of the body functions, never being allowed to eat or drink, no one being allowed to come near the cage. The ants and flies became something awful. The stink of death soon came. And my wife and I and all the village witnessed the starvation and agony and death of our son in that cage."

The man told me that he and his wife waited until late one night, many days after the death of their son, and then escaped across the frontier, and came on down to the village of Muong Sing. I asked the man to come to my house and I gave him some tea. He said something which I put into my notes. He said, "In our village the people are nothing but bricks in the wall of the state." I remembered that in America our state exists only of the people and by the people and for the people.

As the months went on, we suddenly realized that it was almost Christmas time. A few days before Christmas, a plane flew in with dozens of packages of Christmas gifts that had been sent by foresighted people. They probably mailed them sometime in June. The amusing thing was that Christmas gifts continued to come in up to the following Easter. On Easter we had a fake Christmas tree on our piano; on the Fourth of July we received some chocolate Easter eggs. This is how it is in anachronistic Asia.

I do not believe in days off. My crew works every day, all day. Every six months I might give them a week or ten days off, but there are no Saturday afternoons or Sundays off. When a child is brought to us hideously mauled by a tiger, how can we close the hospital and say, "No work today." Hospitals and doctors in America can't do this, nor can we in Muong Sing.

I did, however, give half a day's vacation at Christmas. All during the following year when the boys would ask for a day off, I would say: "Why, I gave you guys a half-day off last year."

On Christmas we had all of our staff over for a lunch and we attached to this lunch all of the elegance of Christmas Day at home. The meal was served buffet style, because there were not enough chairs for everybody. We sat on the porch, on the steps, on the table, and on the bed platform, eating and laughing. We explained the American Christmas. We explained the religious significance of Christmas implicit in the very word itself. No doubt the Communists might make grist out of this for their propaganda mill and say, "You see, Dooley is a Jesuit in disguise."

We drank champagne we had bought in Bangkok months before. We cooled it and drank out of coffee mugs. Chai sipped the champagne, and not liking its taste, he spat it out on the floor. Then he apologized for spitting on the floor, but not for spitting the champagne. Everyone had a grand time and all of the gifts we received we gave to our students. Each was individually wrapped and the ribbons and colored papers were just as much a part of the gift as were the T-shirts, sweaters and candy.

All of our Lao student staff agreed they like this custom of the West very much. Ngoan said that he certainly hoped he could live in America for a while and then he could enjoy both Thai Dam holidays and American holidays. We just couldn't tell him that most cities in America do not celebrate the Thai Dam holidays.

I had a task to do on Christmas Day. I was asked by radio

station KMOX of St. Louis to send a Christmas message to America from the Kingdom of a Million Elephants. Into a tape recorder I was to speak a message that would be played on the radio for all America. What could I say? How could I take the huge emotions and thoughts that were in my heart and in neat, clipped and precise form put them into a few minutes? I had too many thoughts, but I went ahead and into my battery-run tape-recorder I tried to express in fragile words our feelings on that Christmas night in the high valley of Muong Sing:

"This is Dr. Tom Dooley speaking to you from half a world away. I know you will not hear this message during the Christmas season, but I believe that the spirit of Christmas throughout the whole world lasts more than just the days around December 25th. I think the Christmas spirit should last each day, each week, each month, each year of all our lives. So what I want to say to you tonight, even though it may be the end of January when you hear me, is this: Christmas is a timeless thing.

"I have a very beautiful card in front of me that was sent to me from Rome. It expresses my feelings towards Christmas better than I could ever do with my own faint breath of talent. Let me read to you my Christmas wish, my Christmas hope, my Christmas thought:

> It is a good thing to observe Christmas Day but it is better to hold the spirit of Christmas through the year. To hold it helps one to feel the supremacy of the common life over the individual life. It reminds a man to set his own little watch now and then by the great clock of humanity which runs on sun time. There is a better thing than the observance of Christmas Day and this is, keeping Christmas. Are you willing to forget what you have done for other people and to remember what other people have done for you? Are you willing to ignore what the world owes to

you and to think of what you owe to the world? To put your rights in the background and your duties in the middle distance and your chances to do a little more than your duty in the foreground? Arc you willing to see that your fellowmen are just as real as you are and try to look beyond their faces into their hearts, hungry for joy?

Are you willing to admit that probably the only good reason for your existence is not what you are going to get out of life but what you are going to put into it? To close your book of complaints against the management of the Universe and to look around for a place where you can sow a few seeds of happiness? Are you willing to do these things even for a day? Then you can keep Christmas.

Are you willing to stoop down and consider the needs and the desires of little children, to remember the weakness and loneliness of people who are growing old, to stop asking how much your friends love you and ask yourself whether you love them or not? Are you willing to bear in mind the things that other people have to bear in their hearts? To try to understand what those who live in the same house with you really want, without waiting for them to tell you? Are you willing to trim your lamp so that it will give more light and less smoke and to carry it in front so that your shadow will fall behind you? Are you willing to make a grave for your ugly thoughts and a garden for your kindly feelings with the gates wide open? Are you willing to do these things even for a day? Then you can keep Christmas. Are you willing to believe that love is the strongest thing in the world, stronger than hate, stronger than evil, stronger than death? And that the Blessed Life which began in Bethlehem over nineteen hundred years ago is the image and brightness of eternal love? Then you can keep Christmas, and if you keep it for a day why not keep it always.

"From Africa, Europe, Sweden, India, from Taipai, Viet Nam, Indonesia, and from all over America we have received Christmas cards this year. These cards have come here to the mountain valley of Muong Sing and the cards all cry the same thought. In this season there is a great unity —a unity of the world, of all races, of all faiths. There is a unity of Protestant, of Jew, of Catholic, of Mohammedan, of

Buddhist. They all unite in this spirit. Why? Why can't this same battered, beaten world unite in a newer, firmer, more meaningful reaffirmation of the splendid basic truths of this Universe? The truth that the brotherhood of man exists as certainly as does the Fatherhood of God. The truth that service to humanity is the greatest work of all.

"At Bandung, several years ago, President Sukarno said that great chasms yawned between nations and groups of nations. Our unhappy world is torn and tortured and the people of all countries walk in fear, lest through no fault of theirs the dogs of war are unchained once again. The life of man today is corroded and made bitter by fear, fear of the future, fear of the hydrogen bomb, fear of an enemy, fear of an ideology. Perhaps this fear is greater than the danger itself because it is fear which drives men to act foolishly, to act thoughtlessly, to act dangerously.

"We know the danger. We know the danger in this era of time and in this area of Asia. We know the leaders of Soviet and Red Chinese communism, the leaders of these nations who denounce God, who despise freedom, who deny individual rights, who exalt treachery, who counsel deceit, who practice terror and intimidation and torture as part of their day's work; who have everywhere possible exterminated every human being in any human institution that has opposed them. We know that Communism has acknowledged as its supreme mission in life the destruction of the last vestiges of our way of life.

"We have also learned something of the new young nations of Asia. We have learned that they are stirring and trying to find a new place in the sun. I have walked with the people of these nations. I have eaten with their princes and in their village huts. I have argued with these voices in the world, with the voices of people who are destined to have a lot more to say about their future than they ever had in the past. I have sensed and known the bitterness, the confusion, the resentfulness. I know now that there stirs in the hearts of many nations in young Asia a new awareness, a new spirit, a new drive. Often it is aimless but it is always stirring, seeking, endeavoring, trying to find that new place under the sun, the Asian sun, the world sun.

"So when Christmas times comes and we think of this day, we should remember that there must be courage now. There must be, because how can there be peace among men if there is no courage among men? We Americans can be courageous without being pugnacious about it. We can stand up bigger than bitterness. We can reject thoughts of revenge. These don't belong in the minds of moral and peaceful men anyway. We can remind ourselves that love is indeed one of the strongest forces on earth. We can remember that we have had to struggle, that the liberty of our forefathers was secured for us through struggle, and that it must be struggled for and resecured by each succeeding generation.

"So, ladies and gentlemen who listen to me back in America, Christmas of 1958 shows to we three men in Laos the unity of a man's spirit, and a potential of this unity. Christmas of 1958 quietly reminds us that the challenge of our era is the godlessness of Communism. Christmas of 1958 re-illuminates for us again the young nations of the world. It sums itself up with the throught that the keynote of 1959 must be for us, each and every one, for America and for all nations of the world, to seek more ways on a world-wide basis, more ways to serve, with courage and love, the humanity of man. This is Tom Dooley signing off from Northern Laos. So long for now."

EIGHT ·

THE HEART OF IT ALL

An ancient Buddhist prayer says, "O Lord Buddha, o Lord of light and love, give my roots rain." For Dooley, Rhine and Davis our mail from America was rain for our roots.

While I was home on my lecture tour I tried to tell high school boys and girls of some of my feelings. I urged them not to be bland and indifferent young boys and girls. I told them not to keep safely within their own confines and customs. They must listen to the rest of the world, to the voices of conflict, the voices of Asia and Africa. They must hear of civilizations that are being torn apart, of peoples dying, of families being uprooted and scattered. They must be exposed to shattering new ideas and strange new forces, the potential that makes their destiny. I tried to point out that most of the people of the world hate them. They must know why they are hated and they must not be afraid of hate. The weapon against that hate, based on ignorance, is love, based on knowledge. Students must look for new distances, reach out for wider horizons.

While I spoke of horizons, they would always bring me down from my pedantic heights with the question, "Well, doctor, what can we, the seventh grade pupils of St. Anthony's, do for you?"

I remember Dr. Schweitzer once telling me, "In America you must only attempt to create awareness, nothing more. Awareness will then act by just being there." I just do not believe this is true amongst the school boys and girls of America. Too many of them bob on waters like boats torn from their moorings. They need direction. They need a clearly marked channel where they can sail. And when put on this channel, or often when the channel is merely indicated, the kids take over the tillers and sail proudly and well. From Hawaii to New York, from Maine to California, from Seattle to Miami, school students had projects for Dooley. They warm the cockles of my heart. Some of these projects:

"Do-It-For-Dr. Dooley Day." (I don't know what they did, but they charged for it, and they sent me a check for several hundred dollars.)

"Eat-A-Hamburger-For-Dr. Dooley Day." This project was explained to me with the following note: "Dear Dr. Dooley, We had an 'eat a hamburger for Dr. Dooley day' and we charged a dollar a hamburger. Doctor, those hamburgers weren't worth a nickel. Enclosed please find $114."

"Shake Rattle and Roll for Dr. Tom." This performance by some young Texans brought in several hundred dollars. And old man Dooley can't rattle or roll even though he does shake a little bit just naturally.

"Popcorn Balls for Dr. Tom." "Money for MEDICO." "Dollars for Dooley." "Duds for Dooley." A group in Detroit had a "Doughnuts-for-Dooley Day." In Hawaii the Junior Chinese Catholic Club had a "Buy-a-Bar Dance" and collected over two tons of soap. (Hawaii must think that Dooley is the dirtiest doctor in Asia.) Not only did these young men and women collect this soap but the president of their club, Fred Luning, then proceeded to con the Navy out of the transportation. We have enough soap to wash almost every child and elephant in Asia.

The flow of gifts is endless. The most stalwart club that has helped me for several years is the Metropolitan Life Insurance Dooley Aid Club. They have sent to us everything from coffee mugs to skivvies. Teresa Gallagher has been their adrenal gland, and is one of these rare girls who understands that along with the prayin' there must also be a little payin'. Not only did she have people praying but she also had them contributing from all around the Metropolitan Life Insurance building. From MLI several thousand dollars came to our high village. And with the money an endless cable of love and help.

The Wilson Club in Bridgeport, Connecticut, sent me the wherewithal for the zinc-lined piano whose story I have already related. They also sent some fine Easter candy which we received in July.

A Mrs. P. G. Spring and Mrs. Leonard sent us a monthly box of cookies from Hawaii, always wonderfully packed and a welcome treat.

Miss Florence Jacko sends us boxes of stuffed animals and toys month after month. However, Miss Jacko made one drastic mistake. She sent us a large box with 40 little tin xylophones. All around the mountain slopes and deep in the valley, from dawn till dusk and back to dawn again, you could hear this endless clinking and clanking of xylophones. Thank you, Miss Jacko, but please—no more xylophones.

One of the most priceless programs through which money and material were earned for us was through a Mr. Lorenz Aggens of the North Shore Country Day School in Winnetka, Illinois. He sent a letter to our New York office which said:

"Here at North Shore Country Day School we are busily engaged in a campaign to collect soap for Dr. Dooley. The students have set the goal themselves, which is equivalent to the combined weights of a selected representative from each grade through 12th. These students climb on one end of a balancing beam. The accumulated soap is piled on the other end. When the total affair is in balance, we will have made it. The total weight is 871 pounds, which is a good deal of soap for just 250 kids. To accomplish this each class is trying to organize a project, the proceeds of which are soap. One class is running a bake sale, another a sweet shop and the three lower grades are having square dances and charging soap for admission. Some of the older boys will have a car rally, and we hope to be able to organize a car wash for some Saturday before the end of the term. If all the kids flunk out of school this year, it will be Dr. Tom's fault."

This letter came to my office on the same day that the Hawaiian soap shipment came. The password in the foothills of the Himalayas in Muong Sing is "Soap, anyone?" But it can be used!

Some kids, ages 4 to 8, baked cookies to help my hospital in Laos. They sold them under the title "Lousy Cookies."

Earl, Dwight and I are simply the hands. The heart is America. I wish that I could extend to everyone personally some of the warmth of the blanket of thanks that comes to us from our villagers. Each one of their gifts adds a stone to the structure of MEDICO and in so doing strengthens the slightly shaky structure of world peace.

My mail ran into thousands of letters each month. Much of it was handled by Gloria Sassano in the New York office of MEDICO. I had to handle a great deal myself. For many years I have followed a personal law which says that I will write ten letters a night. Now I decided to increase it to 14. Many people wrote and said that they would like to join my team. It was impossible to invite all these good young men and women to Laos. If, however, they could pay their plane fares themselves, I was glad to give them a chance to invest some of their humanity in Laos. Such a boy was Jack Regan, of Boston, Massachusetts.

I had met Jack in Boston several times when lecturing there. For a graduation gift his father gave him a trip to Laos. Jack had no medical training whatsoever, nor did he have much mechanical aptitude. However he cheerfully contributed his services in building, chopping wood and working as a general handyman around the compound. Soon he learned to give shots and we utilized him as a corpsman too. Poor Jack, he suffered from any job that happened to be needed. "Jack, build that bear pen, would you please?" "Jack, drive the jeep out to Ban Nam Di and pick up that patient." "Jack, get that thing painted would you? It doesn't look very well." "Jack, put a dressing on that patient and tell him to come back tomorrow."

Such was life in Laos for Jack Regan, and he spent several months with us. One of his greatest contributions to Tom Dooley was his faith. Dwight and Earl were not Catholics, Jack was. As a consequence I had someone with whom to say my nightly rosary. This rosary meant a great deal to me. It was impossible to taste fully the passing moments of our life. There was no time in Laos to pause, one had to keep running. But during the peaceful silence of night those few quiet moments with my rosary seemed to be the only time that I could get completely out of myself and be tranquil.

Jack was quick to learn the philosophy of our program. He did not agree with many things when he first got there. He thought we were too simple, too down to earth, as indeed we were. We had none of the more complicated things of modern life. He soon realized that to be effective in Asia a program must have an answer expressed in Asian terms and values. What we were trying to do on a medical level was something that the villagers could easily understand. And when they understood it, they were happy.

There are many who bless our work, but there are also some who criticize it. Several of the critics of what we are trying to do are in high places; their main criticism of our work is that we are short-ranged. I believe basically as follows: we should go to places to which we are asked, build and stock a small hospital, train the villagers to run the hospital on a simple level, and after a few years—two, three or four—turn the hospital over to the host governments. Though each MEDICO team is a little different, most of them are based on this concept. The host government where each MEDICO team is situated must furnish many things. In Laos all of the indigenous salaries of my personnel, students and interpreters, cook and housemen are paid by the Lao Minister of Finance. I have *carte blanche* for the Lao medical warehouse and some thirty or forty per cent of my supplies come from them monthly. The Lao Government furnishes all internal transportation and of course Customs-free entry. Whenever I'm in need of things such as cement or metal roofing I get this from the Lao Government. The Lao Government on a local level gives me my working parties and our mason, carpenter and any help we ever need here. We have a medical evacuation program set up with the Ministry of Health so that if anybody at the Nam Tha hospital cannot be treated by the Lao staff there he can be flown to us in Muong Sing on a Government requisition.

When I first heard of the formation of the Woman's Division of the Lao Red Cross I wrote them a letter and asked for blankets for my hospital. They were delighted and immediately dispatched 100 brand new blankets. I thanked them, pointing out that I believe Lao aiding the Lao is much better than the Americans aiding the Lao. The hospital at Muong Sing is *not* an American hospital. Rather it is a Lao hospital that Americans are running for a while.

The powerful and sometimes immaculate dispensers of American aid believe that my philosophy is short-sighted. They claim that the villages cannot maintain what I build. I admit they perhaps cannot maintain it at my level, but I am confident that they can at a lesser level which is still superbly higher than the medical level of the area. I have had many, many visitors to my hospital from Washington. Most of them arrive with that chip on their shoulder, looking around to find the weak spots. Among "jungle doctors" the world over adaption to the environment in an effort to maintain simplicity is the keynote of survival.

Nam Tha furnished my critics a chance to find grist for their mills. Two years earlier we had come to Nam Tha with my former team and had started a hospital. We trained the personnel to a certain level, then turned the hospital over to the Lao Government on our departure at the end of 1957. The Lao Government then sent a "doctor" to the area. There are only two M.D.'s by international standards in the Kingdom of Laos, but there are some 25 *médecins indochinois*. These men have not had the equivalent training of an international M.D. At the end of their *lycée*, which is second-year high school (the highest education that France left to this kingdom after almost a century of occupation), these students went to Cambodia or to Hanoi. They pursued a four-year course of medicine which by our educational system in America would merely be two years of high school and two years of college. They were then diploma-ed as "doctors." I know many of these *médecins indochinois* and some of them are excellent men, but unfortunately not all of them are.

The one who was sent to take over my hospital was a young man. As sometimes happens when young men are taken from villages for education, in returning to their village they feel haughty and superior. So it was with this young man. He felt that, having become a *médecin indochinois*, he should live in the capital and have life a little easier. He did not like being rusticated in the villages of the north.

As soon as I returned to Laos in 1958, I was told how "terrible" the situation was at Nam Tha. The USOM representatives who handle American foreign aid told me with delight and glee how inadequate the *médecin indochinois* at Nam That was, how poorly the hospital was being run, and how only 30 or so patients were being seen a day. If they had remembered that before we got there, no patients were seen, they would have to admit that 30 a day was an improvement, even though less than the 100 a day we had seen.

I was urged by all of the USOM types (a) to go to Nam Tha and straighten that situation up, or (b) to return to Nam Tha and resume my work. I refused. I claimed that I had begun this program and turned it over to the Lao Government. It was a Lao responsibility and a Lao problem, and none of my business. I had no right to go stomping into the area and demanding this and that.

Instead, we went and built our new hospital at Muong Sing. After a few weeks I dropped down to Nam Tha for a visit. All of my former students came to me and complained about the doctor, pointing out how inadequate he was, how he came to work late, how he kept all the medicines locked up so that they could not take care of people, how all the minor surgical instruments and sutures that the student staff knew how to utilize were unavailable because they too were locked up. I told them, as I had told the Americans, that I could do nothing about it and suggested that they go to their own Government representatives and complain. I suggested that every time a Lao official came up, some member of the community should speak to him about this unhappy situation.

I reminded the "doctor" in front of his staff that the Lao government had established an evacuation program. If ever there were a patient with a surgical problem or a disease that he did not feel capable of handling, he should fly him to me at Muong Sing. The doctor agreed, smiling broadly. And that was all he ever did, smile broadly.

This "doctor" at Nam Tha was also Chief of Medical Affairs in the province, and my hospital at Muong Sing came under him administratively. On several occasions I was obliged to send a military telegram to ask permission for a plane ticket, or a working party, or some quite minor matter. Several times he refused me flatly. But there was nothing I could do. I was an invited guest in this foreign land, and I was not going to make the kind of mistake that too often is the white man's error in Asia. I was not about to storm around criticizing, complaining, and demanding.

I believed that if enough Lao heard about Nam Tha they would finally do something. Indeed they did. Many months later when I was in the capital the Minister of Social Welfare and Health, Colonel Sananikone, called me and said, "Thanh Mo America, what is the trouble up at Nam Tha?" I was delighted that he had asked me and I related the whole messy situation to him. He said that he would like to act immediately but that he had no one else to send up there. I suggested that he take one of my male nurses, a graduate of the school in Vientiane, and send him to Nam Tha, pointing out that then there would be superb collaboration between Muong Sing and Nam Tha. Colonel Sananikone agreed; a few weeks later the doctor was transferred and my man ordered to Nam Tha. We were all pleased, especially my nurse who was then promoted to Chief of Medical Affairs for the province. My former assistant was very cooperative about giving me permission to buy a plane ticket.

Under the tutelage of the new man, the young men and women at Nam Tha pitched into things with a vitality that I remembered them as having possessed. Earl and Dwight at various intervals have visited the Nam Tha hospital and are delighted with the way that the students are carrying on. The province is happier, we are able to send down more medicine and aid, and they in turn send us patients that they feel they cannot handle. Because we treat this as routine, there is never any loss of face. As for certain criticisms of the ability of the crew at Nam Tha I can only say what I always say: "In America doctors run 20th century hospitals. In Asia I run a 19th century hospital. Upon my departure the hospital may drop to the 18th century. This is fine, because previously the tribes in the high valleys lived, medically speaking, in the 15th century."

On two of our visits to Nam Tha, we continued on down the Nam Tha River to a village called Ban Houei Sai, repeating the river trip that I had made in the fall of 1957. We made this *pirogue* trip twice in December, 1958 and later in February, 1959. This February trip became a turning-point in my whole destiny.

At first we were reluctant to make the river trip in February because there were rumblings of war again in the Kingdom of A Million Elephants. We had heard radio reports of guerilla murders and of many areas where small infiltrations and skirmishes were taking place. We knew that the Communists had been kicked out of the coalition government and the new pro-Western government of Premier Phoui Sananikone was an honest one, yet still shaky.

Communism had not seized any major chunk of land for several years in this part of the world, and it looked as though there were going to be another try. Therefore we were apprehensive about starting out on a 15-day river trip in the most distant corner of Asia. Some of the territory through which we would pass is territory where there had been former battles. We talked to the Chief of the Military and to the Ministry of Health; they said that they would furnish us with police and military protection. They thought this would be adequate, though they were reluctant themselves to accept any kind of responsibility for us. I always smile when people want to "accept responsibility for Dooley." As I see it, only Dooley is responsible for Dooley.

The people whose villages crouch along the sides of the Nam Tha River in north Laos are some of the most wretched, sick and diseased people I have ever seen. They had nothing in the way of medicines, only the brews concocted by the witch doctor.

The allegiance of these people to their central royal government was a tenuous thing. This royal government, as an independent unit, has existed in name since the 1949 treaty of acceptance into the French Union. But this was in name only. In actuality the Geneva Treaty in 1954 gave birth to a really free government. The people recognize the King and local important officials; but without communication, and the woeful lack of schools, they have little knowledge of the government which guides their country—or even about the country itself. Just the presence of the military men standing guard for us was a complete reverse of the customary situation of Westerner with Asian. I felt it essential to our task in Laos to take our medical aid to these villages as often as possible. As we were sent and supported by the Lao government, there was a good political overtone to the trip. The existence of unrest there increased the need for our river trip in February, 1959.

Earl stayed in Muong Sing this second trip, while Dwight, Chai, Ngoan and several military corpsmen came along with me. We did a great deal of planning, separation of equipment, and calculation of how much to take with us. The Lao Government had sent us an Army DC-3 and we flew all our gear, including nearly 1000 pounds of medicine, to Nam Tha.

In the few days we spent there, walking around Nam Tha flooded my mind with memories. There is the hut where we had that difficult delivery; here a place where a child died of smallpox; here the house of the school teacher who was our best English student; here we worked all night to save a burnt child; there is where the villagers gave a dance for us; here is where we all lived and laughed and loved.

Returning was a very nostalgic thing. All of our former nurses gave a big party for us. Now that my man from Muong Sing was in charge, all was going well. I think that the most important component of a hospital is not lavish air-conditioning, nor electricity, nor fancy electronic paraphernalia, but rather compassion. Nam Tha, completely maintained and financed by the Lao Government, had plenty of this.

Some former students of ours lived in our old house in Nam Tha. I couldn't help noticing that our interior decorating scheme was changed markedly. Where Eisenhower's picture had hung, there was now the photo of the King of

Laos, and our kelly-green paint had turned a dusty green-brown. However, the old house flooded our minds with memories of Johnny and Pete and Denny and Bob and Dammit too. We had been sitting on the porch only a few minutes, when visitors began to arrive.

Remember Ion, the lad who had been so hideously burned? He was the boy we had found in a dirty hovel of a hut, his burned and charred flesh covered with maggots. Remember how he was in our hospital for many months in 1957? He's quite a grown-up lad now, well healed, and he smiles more enchantingly than ever before. His picture is on the cover of *The Edge of Tomorrow*. As usual he brought me a gift, just as he had done every day two years ago. His gift was three eggs and a coconut.

Old Maggie, the village sorceress, dropped in for a chit-chat. I really cannot say that we discussed any of the new antibiotics on the pharmaceutical market, but we did have a good reunion. She had the same crummy towel wrapped around her head as she had two years ago. I gave her a can of shaving cream for a present. No, she doesn't shave but the soap comes out of the aerosol in such a magic way, and if she puts this on wounds it will be a lot more sanitary than her own beetle-juice-cock's-blood-uric-acid compound.

I was glad to find out that the local whisky at Nam Tha had improved slightly. It was still as powerful as ever but some of the kerosene taste had left. If you drop a little on your skin, it blisters.

Nam Tha now boasted four jeeps and a truck and one caterpillar tractor, the last having been parachuted in. American aid was building a road from Nam Tha to Muong Sing. Every vehicle to be used on this road will have to be flown in.

A neighboring tribal village, the Dam village of Ban Nam

Mieng, asked if we would come over for a banquet. I used the word "banquet" very loosely. I believe that at one time or another every villager from Ban Nam Mieng had been in my clinic at Nam Tha. When they heard that their Thanh Mo America had returned, they insisted on entertaining us. We accepted. I have always believed that to get nearer to the heart of Asia, Americans must use their own heart more. But in Ban Nam Mieng it has been proven that occasionally one has to use his digestive tract as well.

On long, low tables some twenty-five feet in length many wooden bowls of food had been laid out for us. The dinner was given in the house of the Tassieng, or village chief. They had palm branches and leaves along the floor with silver bowls and planks of wood. Various assorted pieces of meat, vegetables and greens were set on top of leaves. The food represented every imaginable kind of thing to eat, plus a few unimaginable. There were pig's feet, bat wings, tripe, fish sauces, buffalo steaks, and various herbs, sweet-smelling and otherwise. There were some fetid cuts of meat and an anemic, limp-looking salad that we jokingly call "a dysentery dish." There were several bowls of raw frogs, assorted insects, fried beetles, tubers, cooked bark and roots, and some emaciated sparrow carcasses. But there was one large, lovely dish, the masterpiece of the evening. This hand-hammered silver bowl, set in the middle of the table, crowned the whole repast. It was full of warm, freshly congealed pig's blood. That's right, pig's blood!

We stayed on late, enjoying the warm comradeship of old friends. Villagers brought us the babies I had delivered a year or two ago. Former surgical patients dropped in to the chief's hut to show me how well their scars had healed or their bones knit. Many asked about my former team, Johnny and Bob; many wanted to know whether Pete had put on any weight. The visit was just like the homecoming of any country doctor in America when he goes to a county fair. A doctor's life lights up when he sees his former patients in good health. He helped them regain it, and his inner joy is quiet and good.

The next day we spent making the final arrangements for our trip. The governor had already called for the long dugout canoes, *pirogues.* They were waiting for us down on the river bank. On the following day, we loaded into four *pirogues.* We started about dawn. We now had over 1,000 pounds of medicines, plus bedding rolls, knapsacks, mosquito nettings, foot lockers full of cooking gear, canned foods and assorted bric-a-brac. Three police guards came along with their packs and rifles. Three of my Lao military student corpsmen came: Deng, Panh and Dam. Each of these boys had his pack and a basket of glutinous rice. Chai, my interpreter, had his gear (and, I suspect, a little herbal medicine). We looked more like an invasion party in war than a medical team in peace.

Because of problems similar to those encountered by any family leaving for a Sunday picnic, we didn't really get shoved off until noon. Just as we pushed off, Dwight gingerly opened up his shirt and held up a six-pound baby monkey that someone at Nam Tha had given to him. He was afraid to show it to me until we got out on the river, in case Dooley's humanitarian instinct would demand that the animal be released rather than brought along. "O.K. We have one more passenger," I said. "At least he doesn't have a full pack of gear."

Just a few minutes out of Nam Tha we hit our first set of rapids. The boat plunged into the center of the stream. It then thudded heavily against the underwater rocks. Water poured into the dugout canoe on each side, thoroughly soaking the seats on the bottom. These canoes, about 30 feet long, are made from huge trees that are halved in center, burned and cut out. They have no motors or outriggers. They capsize very easily, though the villagers keep saying, "Don't worry, doctor, they can't sink." (Little consolation to me with thousands of dollars worth of medicines that *can* sink.) Though the rapids lasted only a few minutes, at each set of them I aged a few years.

The first night we slept in a little splash of a village called Ban Saly. There are only about 100 people who live here and 80 per cent of them were at sick call in the morning. Real illnesses—malaria, tuberculosis, pneumonia, chronic coughs, hookworm anemia and always, always the pathetic pot-bellied children of malnutrition. The people of Laos are not a happy, care-free people. They laugh and smile, but they suffer. Their existence is eked out of this life with great effort, just as their villages are hacked from their savage jungles with great difficulty.

This village story was repeated again and again, day after day for the next twelve days. It was not unlike our work at Muong Sing, but here the misery seemed to be in greater intensity. There was greater desolation and everything seemed to be more difficult.

In most of the villages we saw absolutely no indication of American aid in the north—no wells, no rural sanitation, no posters, no roads, no schoolhouses, no farming techniques, no development programs, none of the things that newly independent nations so badly need.

The fault is not with American aid alone. The fault is not all because of apathy in high places in the Lao government. But I feel that if both parties concerned do not show better results soon, the Communist propaganda may succeed, just because it sounds like "a change," even though they are promising pie in the sky bye and bye, as they accuse us of doing. But while we preach of our good intentions and loudly proclaim our plans, programs and blueprints, the Communists move in amongst the naked masses of people and seize power.

Recently an educational program was opened up under the American Economic Aid Mission. It is training village teachers, and it is superb. We met two Lao teachers on this trip, and they are indicative of real progress. I feel we have to stop thinking of hydroelectric plants, dams, super-highways and vast import-export programs. I think we should work more for objectives within the villagers' capability. We should find out what they want and help them to achieve this.

In these villages there is always hunger. Not the dramatic starvation of famine, but daily privation. One of the greatest medicines that we possess is a protein extract called Meals for Millions. This foundation in Los Angeles has given us over 10,000 pounds, and has pledged 5,000 pounds of this extract for every one of the MEDICO teams around the world. I have seen the spindly-legged, pot-bellied children stand taller and straighter, and become bright-eyed and happier. The people who make and support this program, Meals for Millions, should also stand tall and hold their heads high, for they have exercised the greatest power that God has given to man—they have helped their fellow man.

We did not have to fight a barrier of fear and apprehension. Within five minutes after we climbed out of our canoes, half of the village was helping us unload and carry our boxes to the house of the Chief. We had been in their village before, and were returning as friends. We would sit outdoors before the Chief's house in a large semi-circle, surrounded by our medicines and our students. We tried to maintain a little order in the chaos of the sick call, but the important thing was that we maintained distribution rather than order. I would examine the patients and then they would go down to the next person in line, one of my Asian corpsmen. He would give them their medicines, or they would go to the other end of the line for their shots. I'm sure many people came just to chitchat, and others came to "see the show." But as long as they were there, they might just as well bring up that old backache of theirs.

Dwight's new-found friend, the always-unnamed monkey, was tied to the nearest tree to distract the children and the adults too. They could not understand why we didn't eat the monkey, so young, so succulent, so tender. Fried monkey meat? No, thank you.

There were many things that vividly impressed themselves on my mind on this trip. One was an awareness of God, of the great pattern of the universe, the similarity of all the world, the magnificence of the dense green jungle, the majestic cathedral-like colors of the rain-forest, the rapids and rivers flowing one into another. All this cries of a Creator; this speaks of God. For me it is harder to know God in the tumult of plenty, in city traffic, in giant buildings, in cocktail bars, or riding in a car with a body by Fisher. But just as a maker is stamped on America's product's, so is His stamp on all the universe.

Here was God, even in the decay of the villages, because in the death of yesterday there was a birth of tomorrow. We were very lucky to be in the middle of this mystery and wretchedness. We had seen, known, felt and held great beauty. Yet there was a dull, dreary monotony of misery to all sick-calls. Even beside the river, with its constantly changing panorama, this monotony was all-enveloping. Quickly, all could become over-luxurious, over-green, too dense. The rain-forest trees would seem too high, too majestic. And each night seemed a little more uncomfortable than the night before. Here in its essence was the contrast I had tried to point out to Earl and Dwight many months before beside the pool of the Leper King—magnificence holding misery.

We would pull into a village to spend the night. We could not plan ahead of time, because there was no way of judging how far down the next village was or when we would get there. The people here did not lead any kind of life governed by watches strapped on their wrists. If you asked how far or how long it took to get to the next village, they would just say, "Well, you will get there before the sun sets." Even that, we found, was not always reliable.

When we pulled into the village where we were going to have evening sick call, we held our clinic first and then went down to the river to bathe. Though not really cold in the evenings, it was definitely too chilly for river bathing. Anyway, we never came out feeling very clean. Every day I threatened to abandon my nightly bath (but I had not abandoned it yet). We would then eat a dinner composed of a mixture of canned rations, local chickens, eggs, and anything else we could pick up. The chickens of Laos lead a very independent life; not penned up, they run loose in the village and forage around, and each of them is wiry, tough and brawny. To us, however, they tasted good; we were a hungry crew.

We always slept in the hut of some village Chief. Our nights were not very comfortable. It is strange how the sleeping habits of the Westerner depend upon a mattress of some sort. We become addicted to it. At least I have; I don't care how thin, there must be a mattress between me and the bamboo floor. At Muong Sing we had them, on the river trip we did not.

In several of the villages on the river we saw a disease that I had not seen frequently since Nam Tha. It is the hideous scourge of this area, and it is known as Kwashiorkor. It is a massive protein and vitamin deficiency, and the disease was first found in a tribe called the Akra in Africa. Kwashi is a name meaning "a boy who was born on the seventh day." In Africa Kwashi is as common a name as Tom or John, but it is also used to refer to any country fellow, a simple man, a kwashi. The kwashi of Africa often suffer from malignant malnutrition. But others in the world are hungry too, and Kwashiorkor has become known everywhere as a hated and dreaded disease.

What does the victim of Kwashiorkor look like? A child first becomes peevish, irritable; soon he becomes apathetic, his belly bloats, and he sickens. He then becomes indifferent, shows none of the interests, liveliness, or smiles of childhood. If disturbed, he becomes resentful, but shows no vigor in this resentment. He just becomes listless. He doesn't cry, or laugh, or smile. He shows no response to stimulation. Soon he stops eating completely, and then he dies.

However, this is one of the most easily treated diseases. Mead Johnson gave every MEDICO team a large supply of vitamins and proteins. More important than the vitamins and the proteins is education. It does little good for me to give children the medicines and have them fall right back into the same malnutrition environment due to poor dietary care and ignorance. We educate the parents; we explain patiently and tediously about good diet. The people listen. They are eager to know. They do not want the scourge of Kwashiorkor in their village.

The hospitality of the villagers along the river is a warming thing. Their simplicity is delightful. There's no complexity to their lives. Disease and suffering, yes; but also simplicity and kindness. When we come to a village they come down to the river's edge and present a bowl of flowers to us. Sometimes the girls throw a silken scarf across their shoulders and tie it around their waists, and present to us an offering of eggs and fruit.

My boys and I talked a great deal about fundamental questions. Here we were living with some of the most primitive peoples of the world, but they were all men and women of the same human race. Such questions came to mind as these: Is it true that all men are created equal? Or is it true for only some of them? Is it true that they are all endowed by their Creator with the same inalienable rights, or only some? Is it true that among these rights for all are life, liberty and the pursuit of happiness, or only for some? And doesn't the pursuit of happiness include health? I believe that poverty and malnutrition and wretchedness, which make health impossible, are not God-made, but wholly man-made, but the cure for the scourges, the compassion to want to cure, this also comes from God.

We continued plunging down the river. Seven days, eight days, nine days, ten days. On the eleventh morning the river lurched. Wretchedness, misery, stink, poverty. Southward the mighty Mekong River loomed up before us. Here, in an area of deep swirling water, the small Nam Tha River dumps into the large Mekong.

The Mekong River rises from the high plateaus of Tibet at an altitude of about 15,000 feet. It is over 3,000 miles long. It descends slowly through the Chinese province of Yunnan and then forms a frontier between Laos and Burma and later Laos and Thailand. The river continues south, crosses Cambodia and enters into southern Indo-China. It is a benevolent river. It rises slowly in the rainy season and in Vientiane when it reaches its summit it is 40 feet higher than the dry season height. The river rises and falls slowly. The villagers never have to worry about floods, they do not have to build dikes, they can plant fertile rice and vegetable fields along the banks. The Mekong River is a major artery in this part of the world, as well as a good friend of the villages.

Twenty miles up the Mekong River from its junction with the Nam Tha River is a village called Ban Houei Sai. At Ban Houei Sai there is a border patrol station, a landing strip, and a short-wave radio. By this eleventh day we had dispensed the two boatloads of medicines, and we were able to jam ourselves into one small outboard motor boat and one large canoe. We then began the most difficult task of poling up to Ban Houei Sai. It took the whole of one day and the morning of the following day to cover this distance. The boats go along close to the banks of the river, and the natives put bamboo poles onto the earth and rock, pushing upstream. The canoes that we had used to come down from the village of Nam Tha now returned. It would take them nearly a month to pole their way back up to Nam Tha.

At the end of the first day poling up-river, we were really exhausted. We stopped for the night along the eastern bank of the river, where there was a long bed of sand, with a rapidly rising cliff covered with craggy rocks. About 25 feet almost straight up in this jungle, there was a small village of only a few huts.

Chai and I walked across the sand and climbed up the slope to ask the village Chief if we could stop over night in his area. He said we could, and we started to go down the slope to the canoe where the crew was waiting to unload our gear onto the beach. In coming down the side of the slope, just after stepping down carefully on a precarious rock, I tripped and lost my balance. Head over heels I fell down the cliff, banging my chest and my head, gashing open a small spot behind the hair line, and badly hurting my chest. When I hit bottom, I had to lie doubled up for a few minutes to get my breath.

Chai immediately came down to my side and asked if I was all right. I told him that as soon as I could get my breath I would be, though I had badly skinned and bruised the right side of my chest wall, just below the shoulder. I realized then that my boots were unlaced. We do not wear our boots in the canoes, and I had slipped mine on before getting out without lacing them all the way. Through my own stupidity, I had tripped on the lace of my boot, plunging headlong down this 25-foot drop, bouncing my rib-cage off a few of the rocks. I was really sore.

I did not of course realize it, but that fall was to become a pivotal point in my life.

We arrived in Ban Houei Sai around mid-morning. The landing-strip was large enough for a small single-engine plane. At the radio station I sent a message to the capital requesting the Lao government to send us a plane. I also sent a requisition telegram to the civilian airline, knowing that probably one or the other would not make it.

I sent the messages at 10 o'clock, and we sat on the airfield all that afternoon. No plane. We rolled our bags out and slept on the ground at the airstrip that night. The next morning we started our vigil again. Day two passed and no plane; the third day dawned. This was the morning of the day that I was supposed to be in Vientiane, to speak to several hundred people at the International Community. With a three-day leeway, I thought I couldn't miss. If a plane did not get there by three o'clock, we would not be able to fly to Vientiane by sundown. No flying was then allowed in the Kingdom of Laos at night because there are no airports with lights on the landing-strip.

We wondered whether the war had flared up. Was all of Laos now in the flames of combat? Were no planes allowed to come for us? Would we be isolated and left abandoned in this village? While talking about all this, we heard the distant drone of a motor. At 2:30 in the afternoon, the small plane landed and we clambered aboard as fast as we could.

In the air I glanced down at an opening in the jungle and I could see the Nam Tha River curlicuing between the ranges of mountains and I thought over what we had seen and done in these river villages for the last fifteen days. I thought less about my fall than about other incidents on the trip, but later I was to have good reason to remember it.

NINE · THE HANOI BROADCASTS

Over 14,000 refugees from China had escaped into our valley in the past year. The Communists were furious and proclaimed loudly that Laos was aiding and abetting people to leave China. In order to prevent provocation, the police in our area were ordering the refugees to return to China. We recognized the familiar Red tactics: they wanted border "incidents" in order to justify infiltration and invasion. The simple people who had escaped, fearing they would be ordered back to certain death, invented hunting accidents such as the following.

A young Kha Kho tribesman was brought down from the mountains, carried on a large stretcher. His whole upper left arm had been completely torn away by bullets. The lead had also peppered his belly and chest. His wounded arm, wrapped in monkey-skins and packed with tobacco and dung, was of course highly infected. The muscles had been brutally torn and the main arm vessels lacerated. We gave him antibiotics, vitamins, intravenous infusions of glucose and proteins, anti-malarials, and a complete bath. Then we put him on the operating-table. Dwight gave him sodium pentathol and Earl, in spite of having a mild case of infectious hepatitis, came over to the hospital to assist me in the surgery. We were able to close his arm up, but in a few days the swelling from lymph obstruction tore the suture-line open. A few weeks later we had a visiting surgeon who helped me to do a skin graft. The skin graft had about an 80 per cent "take"; in short, the Kha Kho boy came through all right.

The Kha Kho are a warm and simple people. We became very fond of this boy while he was a patient of ours. He often came to the house and thumbed through picture magazines. His friends gave him a haircut, leaving just a pigtail. He delighted in washing himself several times a day with soap, which was something he had never seen before. We had one interpreter for his dialect who would come over several times a day to visit.

The boy came from the frontier and I was convinced that, in attempting to escape from China, he was shot by the frontier patrol. If he had admitted that he was a refugee, the police would have had to send him back to China. Nevertheless, because of the circumstances of the case, the police had to be brought in and the boy claimed that he had been hunting, had climbed up a tree, and that another hunter had mistaken him for a bear and shot him. I was glad for the boy's sake that the police accepted this story, and it was obvious to me from the nature of the wound that his assailant *was* a hunter—a hunter of escapees on border patrol, who had too good an eye to mistake a man for a bear.

There was much rumor of war now, and foreboding through all the North. Once again it seemed as though the dogs of war were going to be unchained. These border skirmishes along the Vietnam frontier and along the China border were increasing. Radio Hanoi and Radio Peking were becoming more vehement in their attacks on Laos. The broadcasts of Radio Peking are required listening for all who live in China. The same is true of the Vietnamese, who must listen to Radio Hanoi. The refugees tell us that they were harangued hour after hour by speeches, denunciations and propaganda. Over the air the anti-American venom was devastating, with such words as "imperialist" and "colonialist" appearing frequently. Every vacillation of our foreign policy in Washington, every news story about the school situation in Little Rock, every single piece of bad news in the U.S. was instantly exploited by the Communist radio, and more verbal violence was unleashed against the western world.

Never had I heard of a medical program being attacked until the month of March, 1959, although anything that is accomplishing something of value for the Free World is usually attacked in an attempt to destroy its efficacy.

The Communists were accusing us of espionage activities. By shouting day and night about this sort of thing they were creating a certain doubt. If you accuse someone over and over, week after week, month after month, the listener begins to believe what he hears. The repetition induces suspicion and finally belief.

Recently in Vientiane, a Minister himself had said to me, "Dr. Dooley, Radio Peking accuses you of espionage in North Laos."

"That's absurd, isn't it?" I replied.

"You don't work for any agencies of America, do you?"

The mere fact that he added the Lao equivalent of "do you" indicated to me that suspicion was being implanted even in his mind by these radio attacks.

This is exactly the kind of vulnerability the Communists aim for. That is how they could destroy my mission in Laos. If they repeated lies about us long and loud enough, soon the lies might seem like the truth to the government leaders in Laos. The Communist plan was obvious. Why did they want my medical program out of here? Because they are basically opposed to medicine? No. Because they realize that our hospital is helping the free Royal Lao Government to establish itself firmly. At the same time it is helping to unite ties of friendship between the people of Laos and the people of America.

To force this hospital to go home, the Communists would have to fill the Lao Government officials with suspicion that perhaps we are doing more than they are aware of. If we were selling opium or spying or running around with their village women, the Lao government would be alarmed. And if they felt that our presence is a threat to the peace and security of their country, obviously they would be forced to ask us politely to leave. I was sure that the Lao Government realized that the mere fact that the Reds were attacking us was proof positive that our actions were having a good effect. Otherwise they would leave us alone. The very fact that the leaders all the way up in Peking, China, were denouncing our three small buildings indicated that we must be doing something worthwhile.

"U.S. secret agents have established permanent organizations in that area under the guise of performing medical services, of running a village hospital. The United States is plotting to provoke conflict on the China-Lao border with the aim of creating a pretext for armed intervention by the United States and other aggressive blocs, and for dragging Laos step by step into war."

Hearing these things said about us did not in any way make us feel secure or safe. In fact, the broadcasts from Hanoi and Peking added a touch of terror to our days and nights.

Another recent Radio Hanoi broadcast said: "The Lao authorities have been acting in collusion with secret agents and organizations . . . permitting them to use the Muong Sing area of Laos to carry out espionage and sabotage activities against China. They have taken advantage of trade across the border to send special agents into China repeatedly to collect information, spread rumors and create disturbances. . . .

"The above mentioned provocations by Lao authorities . . . in the region of Muong Sing and Nam Tha . . . in the last six months . . . are being done under the guise of a medical team. . . ."

The greatest problem that we had to put up with in our kind of work was loneliness. There was loneliness in Laos, but not of a bitter kind; not the loneliness of dead friendships or lost awareness. Rather we had that strange kind of loneliness that men have who find themselves swinging out beyond the boundaries of normal existence, who find that there suddenly bursts upon their view a fleeting moment of almost devastating awareness. We felt as though we were standing on the mountain peak and had, just for a quick moment, a tremendous view of all the world. This kind of loneliness was a good thing, for it made us more aware, and there was no exhaustion of the spirit.

The dull rounds of our daily work, and its accompanying misery, had a tendency to submerge us. We usually found some small thing to prevent this routine from stifling us, but such escape was never peaceful. Since I started medical school I have had to struggle, first with myself, later with an enemy, and now with both. It seemed that complete tranquility, in my time, was just about the rarest parenthesis in life.

The loneliness that I knew was different from the loneliness of my boys. They both missed their wives and Earl his unseen child. Our relationship as a team was such as would exist on a ship with an officer who was liked but who was nevertheless the Commanding Officer. Earl and Dwight always referred to me as "Dr. Dooley," and there was a "sir" at the end of every sentence. Though we shared a deep bond of comradeship, and a deeper bond of common interest and love of our work, there was nevertheless a kind of wall between us, and also putting up with the erascible burrs of my personality is tough on my crew. I drive them hard. I suppose in many ways Dooley is really tyrannical. Earl and Dwight developed a plan of escape from me. They fixed up a den out of a small room (more like a large broom closest) in the hospital. Every night after dinner they would take a kerosene pressure lamp, the battery-run tape-recorder, and retreat to the Bird Room (so named in honor of a single sad old crow Earl had stuffed). There they were free of Dooley's hyperthyroid totalitarianism. The Bird Room was my crew's inviolate cloister.

We had come to the mountains to do our work. The daily routine of our life in this valley jungle, with its habits and techniques, its daily wretchedness, could make one sink almost into lethargy—until terror struck from across the border and plunged us into fear.

One day Chai and I went to a border village to see a very sick man. While there, we were asked to go down the trail and see two new refugees who had just arrived, one of whom was critically ill. We went to a small grass hut built up on stilts; it was poorly erected, rickety and unstable. Inside we found an old man and his daughter.

The young girl's name was Nung Di. She belonged to the Chinese portion of the Thai Lu tribe, living 50 miles inside China. This girl was lying on her side deep in her own filth, with various herbs and incense around her. She was doubled up in acute agony. When I touched her hand, she trembled like a frightened pup and pulled away from me in fear. Nung Di had a massive infection of the hip joint which had spread to the muscles and tissues of the thigh and leg and onto the abdomen. She was a sick and wretched little girl.

I could not speak her dialect and sent Chai to find someone who could. We instructed him to tell her that she would have to be taken to the hospital immediately so that we could give her anesthesia, incise and drain that leg. Otherwise she would either die, or, if she did not die, would be hideously crippled all her life. I watched her face as the interpreter slowly and softly told her my words. She started to cry and became almost hysterical. I touched her hand and tried to reassure her, but again she pulled away from me and became hysterical. She said she would not go to my hospital. The interpreter again was told to tell her that if she did not, she would die. She said, "I don't care. I will die here. I do not want to die in your hospital."

Other villagers who knew me and our work came to talk to her. They patiently explained to her that our medicines would help, that our hands would heal. She sobbed and whimpered like a beaten dog and she and her father both said, "No, no. We will not go to the hospital at Muong Sing. It is a white man's hospital. It has an American doctor." I went outside and sat on the front ladder of the hut, while the Lao talked to them. I knew that Chai would find out the real reason behind her fear. He explained that it was not the usual reticence. Her fear of the hospital had nothing to do with good and evil spirits, with witchcraft, our biggest competitor. The girl was deathly frightened of the American monsters that she had heard so much about.

In her village of Muong Pun in China, the Communist

commissar had held several hundred hours of lectures about the American monsters. He specifically cited the Dooley-Davis-Rhine hospital program at Muong Sing. He said that we were not medical people at all, but secret agents of America. The Commissar said, "The Americans commit heinous crimes, especially against girls. They inject germs into the bodies of young people." They accused us of brutally beating children who would not take our medicines. They accused us of being corrupt and depraved. They said that we had injected medicines into old people and that they died right away, and that we had crippled many people and had foul plans of hurting more. This little girl had been exposed to this for week after week. No wonder she was afraid to come.

After much talking by all of the villagers, she consented to come to our jeep but only if her father and half a dozen people came with her. I carried her down the stairs myself. Her frail, half-bloated body was trembling terribly. We got her to the hospital and onto the operating-table, though it was quite a task. After a little anesthesia, we drained quarts of purple-green pus from her leg, put her on antibiotics immediately, and the moved her to the ward.

The little girl remained a pathetically frightened wisp for several days until our medicines began to have a marked effect. Her temperature dropped, and as the pain disappeared she realized that she was going to be better.

By this time the eloquent compassion of my crew showed its effect. On the fourth day she and her father broke down and told us why they were so fearful; they were sorry that they had been wrong. They fully realized that the lies were part of anti-American hatred, and we knew that China was plunging such hatred into the hearts and minds of the people of that country. How tragic, how inhumane, how miserable must existence be for those who live under the lies of Red China.

In six surrounding villages around Muong Sing we established sub-stations, run by our Lao military students. Each sub-station consists of a small hut with the minimum amount of medicines. The students work in these areas for a month, coming back to stock in more supplies, and to compare notes with me. Dam or Boun Tung would sit beside me as I was holding sick-call at the hospital and say, "Oh, yes, I had a case similar to that just a few days ago. I find that terramycin is most efficacious." It always amused me that the boys who only a few months ago were on the backs of water-buffalos were now talking as one physician would to another at St. Mary's hospital in downtown St. Louis.

Though the work of these Lao military students might be considered amateurish by American standards, they did have talent and they were improving the health of their respective villages. These intense young corpsmen were sparkling and clean. They were very proud of their newly acquired knowledge. They saw "*meh penh yats*" everywhere and must have possessed a microscopic vision to be able to see "germs" so readily. Earl was teacher for the students of these substations. The students were learning, and Earl was surviving.

One of our favorite patients was a young lad of the Thai Dam tribe, called Tao Koo. Tao Koo was seven years old. He had a scorching fever accompanied by diarrhea several months before he came to us. The family put him in to bed, the village witch-doctor incanted something or other, and within two weeks, on a diet of rice and water, the child developed a bed sore. Within a month this had spread until all the flesh of his lower back and buttocks had sloughed off. Over each bony hip he had a dirty ulcer. He became incontinent and this constant soilage only worsened things. He shrank and withered until he was just a shadow of a child. Finally the father brought him to us in Muong Sing, a three-day walk.

Earl and Dwight immediately took the child to their hearts. They took that little urinoid glob of flesh and washed him with all the tenderness they could muster. With gentle hearts and hands and a little of the grace of God, they treated and dressed his sores. The child showed no reaction. He was too sick, too dulled by pain to respond even to this much compassion. They rigged a special bed for him, tying balloons on the cross-bars and pasting pictures on the wall beside him. They gave him a color book and a little rabbit that squeaked and in the few days of sunlight left before the early monsoon season, they took his bed outside and draped a mosquito net over it and let him lie in the sun. The dressings were removed and the sores were aired.

About a week after admission Tao Koo's eyes, so bleak with dying, began to brighten a little. His terrified father learned how to treat him, how to feed him properly, how to bathe him and tend him without injuring what little good tissue was left. The boys rigged a method so that his incontinence would not soil everything. This wistful little lad, God's compromise between flower and dung, an interval between birth and death, once again began to live. He began to smile and answer questions with a word instead of a whimper. This emaciated skeleton, his withered skin tightly pulled around small bones, was now picking up weight and filling out, and his sores were closing. He was perhaps the happiest and definitely the cleanest boy in Asia.

As the sun set and the boys were putting Tao Koo's bed back in the ward, I would sit on the back steps and watch them. There was an immense, quiet happiness in the faces of my two Americans. There was peace in the faces of the

Asians around the compound. There was much beauty in the purple glow of the sunset over the Burmese hills. There was an extraordinary amount of exertion here, danger, some choking futility, and much loneliness. But there were also these moments in the evening when the chaos and sadness of the day melted into the peaceful silence of the night.

At such moments my mind would embrace much. I remembered that my teachers had taught me that humanity is God on earth. I remembered that a doctor's job is to cure sometimes, to relieve often, to comfort always. I remembered the strong vine of friendship that joined my hospital with all our good people of America. I remembered reading Lincoln's "freedom is for all men in all lands everywhere." I remembered just why we were here. And in watching Earl and Dwight care for that little wisp of a lad I was positive that the human spirit can rise supreme, and that man can develop a feeling of oneness with other men. All beings of blood and breath are brothers, here to help one another.

Maybe the dream of Anne Frank is closer than we know: "Things will change and men become good again and these pitiless days will come to an end and the world will once more know order, rest, and peace."

TEN ·

THE NIGHT THEY BURNED THE MOUNTAIN

The month of May brought the hot, dry season to an end. The jungle though still green was dryer than ever. The stream and gullies were dry, and the wet humid dampness of the jungle was no longer present. Though there were not many changes in the color of the leaves, there was definitely an aridness to the high mountain slopes.

The tribes of the Kha Kho and the Thai Dam now began to prepare for their great planting season, called the Duong Pet. The Duong Pet means the eighth month, since in their calender it is the eighth month, the month when the rice must be planted, the month before the rains begin.

For us Americans it was a most uncomfortable period of time. On one particularly warm night I was vividly aware of how anxiously I was awaiting the coolness of the monsoon season. Though each monsoon season I cursed the rains and the gales, I was now eagerly anticipating the cool wild mornings. The soaking rains would be a relief from the oppressive heat that came at the end of this dry season.

The war scare was worse than ever now, with definite shooting in many areas. The rainy season might slow the war down, because the jungles become impassable during the heavy rains. However, under such conditions the war might also take a twist and increase in intensity and it would certainly be a more difficult war to fight, especially by modern means.

Late one night I was sitting in the main room of our house with a kerosene lamp on the table, my typewriter papers and stacks of unanswered mail around me. My T-shirt was soaked from sweat and the kerosene lamp was hissing at me. Earl and Dwight were asleep in the other room, Ngoan and the Lao were in the room on the left. I was writing to my family and friends in America, but more than ever they seemed distant to me now. I had a vague uncomfortable feeling. I wasn't especially worried about the war, yet on the other hand I feared the poison of China flowing into our valley. I had pain in my right shoulder and chest dating from my fall of several months before. The pain had never eased; in fact, several times I sneaked over to the hospital and took some codein. On that particular night I had a feeling of apprehension that was difficult to describe to myself, more difficult to explain.

The night seemed noisier. I had a sensation that there was activity outside the house, so I took a flashlight and walked out on our front porch. The mountains all around us looked as though they were covered by swarms of lightning bugs. As I looked at these blinking, flickering lights moving in all directions, I thought to myself, "Almost like Japanese lanterns in a parade."

Suddenly as I watched I saw one whole section of the jungle catch on fire. Then more fire. And more fire. Suddenly and almost in a flash the whole mountain slope on the Burmese hill burst into a blinding glare of yellow flames. The flickering lights I had seen were people moving down with torches to set fire to the jungle. I walked out to the field across from our house and a whole panorama opened up—the jungles to my south, north, and east were also aflame. Huge billows of clouds were spraying up from the ground and heading towards the sky.

Oppressive rolls of heat poured down into our valley. I had an almost terrifying feeling. Were these Communists? Burning the jungle down? Aiming at the complete annihilation of our village of Muong Sing? Just a few weeks ago they had completed destroyed a village only a few miles away from us, in retaliation for the village taking refugees from China into their huts. Was this another Communist atrocity?

In a few minutes Earl and Dwight, awakened by the heat, ran to the porch and looked with amazement at the sky and the night on fire. The whole jungle covering the mountains around us was alive with flames. In the bottom of the bowl of the Muong Sing valley it seemed as though all three sides of us were blazing, the yellow flames licking at the clear sky, the smoke rolling higher and higher. Ngoan came out, looked at the mountain slope, then looked at us, and said, "Do not fear, Thanh Mo America, this is the night they burn the mountain."

I then remembered seeing such Maytime fires far off on previous occasions in Laos. But never had the geographical pattern been as close and tight and menacing as now.

For the mountain tribes the last week of the Duong Pet is a time of great feasting and great work. These tribes do not plant their rice in water-paddies, as do those who live in the valley, but rather on the burnt slopes of the mountains. The village sorcerers and astrologists choose the felicitous night, and after several days of feasting the people light their bamboo torches. The legend is that someone lit a fire in this land dynasties before the conquest of Kublai Khan. Since that time there has always been a fire somewhere, in some homes, over some cooking-areas, outside some huts. When a villager wants to light a fire, having no matches, he merely goes to the house of his neighbor with a place of flayed bamboo and steals some fire and takes it to his home. On this night all the mountain tribes had lit torches and had gone up to set the mountain slope on fire. The jungle would burn for several days. Then ashes would cover the slopes of the mountain—blackened ashes, and dead earth. But when the rains came, in a few days, the water on the ashes would make rich, fertilized ground. And in this black scorched earth the tribes would plant their rice roots. From the seedlings would grow their rice—not paddy rice, but poor rice, mountain rice.

Earl, Dwight and I watched the mountain burn for many hours. The strange, vague forboding feeling that I had had in the house seemed all the stronger now. What would become of these mountains and these tribes? What would happen to their kingdom of Laos? Would the flames of Communism conquer it? Would the flames of disease destroy the people? Would there ever be another free May when the people would burn their mountains and plant their rice in this blackened earth?

Finally fatigue completely conquered me. In spite of the heat and the still roaring flames all around, I went to bed. Ngoan had explained that the flames would not come below a certain area because the mountain people had dug trenches as fire stops. I went to bed and slept until dawn came over the scorched mountains. It seemed as though the sorcerers and astrologists were right. Only a few days later, before the earth was even cool, the Nyam Fon came.

Nyam Fon, the season of the rains and monsoons. Back at my University of Notre Dame, this was the season of lilacs. Here it was a time of crashing violence and tropical thunder-storms, of gray, dark and murky days. The tropical night no longer whispered, but roared with a torrent of monsoon rain. The rains lashed the high valley, whipped the palms and frangipangi, and flooded the earth. Clouds piled high, and downpours crashed all day and night.

The magnificent sun rose unseen. Steamy breaks of blue weather came, but with it came bugs, rot, mud, and a foggy sash of sunset. This was the season of Nyam Fon, when the whole earth was sodden. In the breadth of the night's storm, the black bats tumbled and darted, the huge insects brushed and flapped and fluttered about.

It was a season when, more than ever, God was everywhere. We saw Him in the mountains, we saw Him in the air, in the mist, in the morning fog. We heard Him in the monsoon rain on the thatched roof. We saw Him outstretching his arms in the lightning and in the thunder of the Nyam Fon. We saw His hand of life in the wind. Even during the rains the village days went on imperturbably with the same rhythms. The villagers prayed to the gods for more rain, to the lord of thunder and the goddess of lightning. They threw firecrackers up into the air to chase away the evil spirits. They wanted the rain and the wind. Their rice hungered and yearned for it; without it, the rice would die.

The trees across the field from my hospital, always clear to see, were now lost. The mountains rimming the valley, the skies and earth alike, all grew dim and vanished in the tide of gray rain. The noonday's silence of a little while ago became the rustle of the wind. Then the wind hummed, and the hum grew deeper and wilder. Then the sound of thunder, the rain, the wind. The thunder and the lightning crashed and rolled and broke overhead. Around the hospital compound were tall palm-tree tops. Above them the sky was blue and violet and blue and dark and then gray again.

The town of Muong Sing was lovely and hideous at the

same time. It was lovely in its majestic site, a deep green valley with the rain-forested hills around it and the thrusting mountains just beyond it. Our valley was beautiful when the sky was high and clear and the horizon was wide. It was beautiful even when the skies were dark and we were surrounded by the all-protecting gods of strength, the mountains of Muong Sing. But how hideous the village could be in its filth and its squalor, how odorous the close-packed fetid huts. The streets were now a sea of filth and garbage. The wretched of the village hacked out their lung tissues and their lives. Great splotches of red betel could be seen all over the ground. The chickens and pigs and water buffalos and cows roamed loose all around the town. Beauty and hideousness—they were both here at one and the same time.

When the monsoon torrent of water flowed down the mountain slopes, the valley floods and the fields grew rich with jade-green rice. The palm trees bowed to the wind as acolytes bow at the *Confiteor*. The people of our valley were completely the victims of external circumstance. They could not control the rain coming, nor counteract the bacteria that flooded their lives, they did not know how to improve their plows, they lacked so much.

Those of us in the world who have these things must not ignore the essential needs of human nature the world over. I used to think: These people will die of misery. I have learned something, an unpalatable truth: No one ever dies solely of misery. I wondered just how these people would live on. I looked at this tranquil, almost sleepy green jungle and realized that neither the earth nor the bulk of its human inhabitants really know much of what is going on. All humans are in some way incomprehensible. Yet all human beings can be understood—and must be. The effort must be made.

Life continued in the village in spite of the rains. In fact, everyone worked harder at this time of the year. With their broad-brimmed Chinese conical hats, the villagers went out into the flooded paddies and planted their rice. In a few weeks their closely packed rice would be pulled up and spaced in the replanting season. All of the villagers got together and worked in one large communal movement. They sang while they worked and there was a wonderful vitality to the air.

Many came to our hospital for sick-call during this time with sores on their legs because their feet had become shriveled and bloodless from long immersion in their paddy water. Also the fungus skin diseases increased at this time.

We were the only ones that the rains seemed to bother. We were unaccustomed to such incessant downpouring, and built rain ramps connecting our buildings—thatched covered walks so that we could go back and forth without becoming drenched.

The Muong Sing landing strip, though it became sodden, was still useful. Though the strip at Nam Tha could not be used, the Muong Sing landing field could handle small planes the year round. Soon after the rains came, I flew to Vientiane to make a quick trip to Phnom Penh, the capitol of Cambodia. Dr. Emmanuel Voulgaropoulos, head of our Cambodia MEDICO team, had invited me to come down and visit his hospital. At Phnom Penh the chief of the Economic Mission lent me his small plane to fly to the village of Kratie, where Manny has his hospital.

Manny's hospital comes closer to the realization of my dream of MEDICO than any other. The small hospital that we have in Kenya is, I would say, second. We have surgical programs in Jordan and Viet Nam, eye programs in India, dental programs in Africa, but closest to my heart is a village team such as Manny's.

Dr. Manny was a 28-year-old bachelor when he came to join MEDICO in December, 1958. Soon after his arrival in Kratie he sent for his fiancée and, for the first time in the ancient history of Cambodia, an American wedding was held. The Governor of the Province first gave Rose away in a Buddhist ceremony, and Rose wore the full costume of the ancient Khmer wedding ceremony. After this ceremony had been conducted with all the ancient pomp and circumstance, a smaller Christian ceremony was held. The whole Kingdom of Cambodia had heard about this American and his bride being married according to the customs of their country, and they loved it.

Manny had with him two young American corpsmen. One of them was a former Navy corpsman, Tony Jagger, which pleased this old salt's heart. Their hospital, a little larger than mine, was located in a large city, with electricity and running water, though primitive and spasmodic. There was a road running through this city connecting with the capital in a murderous 12-hour drive.

Manny was working in close cooperation with the Cambodia government, and although he was having to surmount many obstacles, this was simply part of his occupational hazards. He was doing a wonderful job and his heart had found its mooring in his work. The touch of a woman was very easy to see—curtains on the windows, flowers in the vases, a little study fixed up over the main clinic. Maybe there is something to this connubial bliss.

While I was in Cambodia I heard a very beautiful legend. In origin it belongs to Viet Nam, but it is known and loved throughout all of Indo-China. It is a story of the season of Nyam Fon, and the legend goes like this: Once upon a time, long ago, there lived a very rich king, who had a beautiful daughter. Many young princes came from neighboring countries to beg for her hand, but the king refused them all. One day two handsome young men happened to arrive at the palace at the same time. The first introduced himself as the god of the Mountain, the other as the god of Water. The king's embarrassment was great. Here were two suitors for his daughter's hand, equally handsome, equally rich, and equally powerful. What would the old king do? After much thought, he said, "I will give my daughter's hand to the prince who arrives first on the morrow with the most exotic and fabulous of wedding gifts."

The next day the god of the Mountains arrived first, bringing, silver, gold, ivory and jade. True to his promise, the king gave him his daughter, even though the god of Water had not yet appeared. The couple then left immediately to go to the high mountain castle for their honeymoon. When the other suitor arrived, with even more magnificent gifts, the princess was gone. The god of Water was furious and swore to the blue sky above and to the black earth below that he would win back this lovely young princess. He would wage war against the Mountain. And so the battle began. The god of Water amassed all of his powers to wage war.

First, the elements burst forth, the skies opened up, and rain pelted the earth mercilessly. Tidal waves and floods and typhoons and tornados devasted enormous areas. Amidst all this fury the sea fauna were suddenly turned into soldiers and marched in huge columns to the fortress of the god of the Mountain. The god of the Mountain had power no less great. He transformed all the highland fauna of his mountain into warriors, and turned the stones into white elephants. Dreadful battles took place, and the number of casualties in this war of the gods was tremendous. The damage to the fields of the ancient kingdom was incalulable, for the war dragged on for years and years. Finally the god of the Mountain defeated the god of Water. The latter was forced to withdraw his forces into the sea and the sky. However, he bore with him a grudge and a vow of vengeance that has never left his heart. Every year since that time, the god of Water returns to earth. He floods and thunders and plagues the people of the mountains in an attempt to win the lovely princess. And ever since that first battle, the season when the god of Water returns is called Nyam Fon.

I returned to Laos in a few days, and they were sick days for me. We have a tremendous amount of malaria in our territory of Northern Laos and we take malaria suppressives weekly. When I went to visit Manny in Cambodia I did not take a suppressive; I forgot it. When I returned to Laos I spent the night at the house of Hank Miller. We talked of the war problems, and I mentioned my aching body. I felt quite bad that night, with much generalized fatigue. I thought it was simply because I grow old. The next morning I realized that I had a blazing temperature. I was due to fly out at dawn and I preferred to be sick at my own hospital rather than in the capitol.

I climbed into the plane and had the most awful trip of my life. Every little bump, every little air pocket was excruciating. I thought my head would split into pieces. When I arrived, the boys came out in the jeep to meet me and made some comment like "My gosh, you look like hell, Doctor." I agreed with them wholeheartedly, climbed into the jeep, and we rolled into town, each bump pushing me a little bit closer to the brink of death. Or so it seemed.

By the time I got to the house it was obvious that I was having a first-class malaria attack, complete with chills and 105 degrees of fever. I took the malaria medicines and went right to bed, with half of my hospital staff around to help, aid and succor me. Never was a patient so overtreated as the boss when he got sick. Twenty-four hours in bed and the fever was gone and the chills had stopped. Although I felt tremendously exhausted, I was able to go back to work. I did not get malaria from Manny; it was evidently in my bloodstream when I flew down and the incubation period elapsed while I was in Cambodia. But from that day on we preferred to blame the kingdom of Cambodia for Dooley's malaria.

While passing through the capitol of Laos once again I heard more of war; more skirmishes, more shootings. It looked as though along with the burning of the mountains, the land of Laos might be thoroughly burned by the flames of war.

During the month of June the pain in my chest increased. A lump on my upper chest was getting larger, and had increased from the size of a pea almost to that of a golf ball. My arm ached so badly that I did not play the piano anymore at night. One day, driving the jeep with Chai in the back seat, I had to ask him to lean forward and massage my neck and back because it hurt so much to keep my arm lifted. I thought the lump must be a large sebaceous cyst or a boil that was growing rapidly in size and affecting the nerves and muscles of my chest. Or maybe this was a deep bone bruise, with a bloodclot below the bruise, pressing on tender nerves of the rib cage.

Sometimes it even hurt when I took a deep breath, a stabbing kind of pain into my lung. Some years back I had been badly clobbered on the chest by some angry people of North Viet Nam. Every once in awhile I had vague aching pains in my chest. Was this a left-over of that incident of many years ago, its pain accentuated by the recent fall? While I was at Hank Miller's house in the capitol, he noticed the lump under my T-shirt and asked about it. I jokingly said, "Oh don't worry, Hank, it's just cancer of the lung."

One day in July, during Nyam Fon, the clouds unexpectedly cleared and the sun burst forth in a blinding flash. Almost instantaneously we heard the small roar of a twin-engine airplane and ran out of the clinic yelling, "*Hua bin, hua bin, hua bin,*" (which, as your ears should tell you, means "airplane"). It was good to see that the plane had an American flag on it. We all drove with the jeep out through the water and the mud to the landing strip. Out of the plane stepped an old friend of mine from Solvang, California, Doctor Bill Van Valin. Years ago Bill had promised that he would come and visit my hospital someday and give me a hand with surgery. Now, during the height of the wet season, when the North was consumed in a war, Bill Van Valin blithely arrived in Laos to spend a week.

One of the first things I asked Dr. Van to do was to take a look at my chest. It was now causing me quite a good deal of pain. He saw the lump and immediately suggested that he remove it surgically, agreeing with my pre-operative diagnosis of a rapidly growing sebaceous cyst. The next afternoon, in an almost joking manner, we went to the hospital and I climbed up on the operating-table. Several of my students thought that this was a very funny moment and had many comments to make, such as: "Thanh Mo America himself is getting operated on, instead of doing the operating." "Do you want me to call the witch doctor?" "Lie still, doctor, it won't hurt." Chai leaned over me and moaned and groaned and made comments in Lao while the girls walked in and out of the room smiling.

All the while Dr. Van was busily opening up the skin of

my chest to remove the lesion. I remember now in retrospect the cloudy look that came across his face when he finally got down to the tumor itself. Lying as I was I could not see what he was removing. It was not until he finished and I saw the tumor that I said, "It's jet black, Van?" He said, "Yes, it is."

After my chest wall was sutured we examined the tumor more closely. It was hard, circumscribed, and completely black. There is only one tumor that is jet black. I was not in the least concerned that this was melanoma, truthfully believing the tumor had something to do with a fall, perhaps an old, hardened and partially calcified blood clot. Van agreed with me but was very insistent that the tumor be taken to a hospital in Bangkok for analysis.

He asked me if I had any formalin. I laughed and said, "I should say not, doctor. Do you think you're at the National Institute of Health? If you want to preserve that tumor you will have to be content with just old 90 per cent alcohol." He smiled and said, "No. We must get formalin." Earl came to the rescue and went to his Bird Room and brought back a bottle that he was using in his taxidermy work. Doctor Van prepared a solution of the proper strength and put part of the tumor into the bottle. He would take it with him when he left Muong Sing. In Bangkok there was a large Seventh Day Adventist hospital with a superb pathologist, and Van would have my tumor examined there.

I dismissed the thought of cancer from my mind, and plunged back into my work. Being a doctor with a heavy patient load and a war on my mind, I really didn't have much time for negative thinking. And yet, after a night of good sleep with drugs, the area still hurt plenty.

I was awakened a little after dawn by the work that I was put on this earth to do. A villager had come to take me to Ban Ting That. The chieftan of the village had sent him to say that there was a man who was terribly sick, so sick that he could not allow the man to stay in the village. He had built a thatched lean-to in the field, and put the man in it. With the rest of the symptoms, this sounded very serious to us, like cholera. We climbed into the jeep to splash our way down the soggy trail to the village of Ban Ting That.

In the field outside of the village we found the hut. Not even a hut, really, just four pieces of thatch on a two-foot high wooden frame. Underneath this frame was the most wretched-looking human I had ever seen. The man was desperately sick and was covered with his own excrement. He had a severe infection of the lungs. He was foul-smelling and as he inhaled and exhaled there was a rattling in his chest, a death rattle. His eyes were glazed and the opium gourd on his side indicated to us that he had been taking a great deal in the past days. He was completely dehydrated and responded very sluggishly to even the most violent stimulation. I was seized by a sudden urge to leave the man there and let him die. What could we possibly do for him in such a filthy state? But this was wrong. A doctor shouldn't feel this way. My business is wretchedness, but he was the most disgusting human I have ever seen in my life. We baptized him immediately as I was sure he would die. Ngoan and I picked him up and carried him over to our jeep.

We drove to Muong Sing and were surprised to find he survived the thirty-minute trip. We carried him in to the dressing table and all of my staff pitched in and helped clean him up. We burned his clothes and washed him over and over again until he was clean. Having some guilt about my original feelings towards the man, I bent over backwards to give him full attention every day. We tried to get him to walk, to get him to eat, to get him to breathe deeply. Only after four days did he begin to respond at all and then he began to beg for his opium pipe. He was a hopeless, helpless addict. I started giving him some morphine but soon realized that we could not support him on morphine alone. On the fifth day I withdrew the morphine. We found him dead in bed on the sixth.

We had a little boy in the hospital at this time, a boy whose name was Thai Noi. His brightness helped to offset the sadness of the man's death. Although he was about nine years old, he looked like a withered up little boy of five. He had a huge bladder stone that had taken everything out of his life. He was never able to put on weight, to grow strong, and was constantly racked with kidney infections. We surgically removed the stone, about the size and weight of a golf ball. He convalesced well but when we removed the stitches he developed a fistula. We re-operated on him a second time, attempting to close the fistula, but were unsuccessful. He stayed on at the hospital for many weeks on protein extracts and vitamins and soon the wound healed up and the fistula closed.

Thai Noi's round big eyes grew brighter and cheerier and he put on weight. Soon we had him working around the hospital to earn his living and his father became one of our chief water-carriers; we are constantly carrying water from the well to the hospital and the house. Thai Noi used to come and sit in our house and talk with Ngoan, as they were both of the same tribe. He became very much an intimate part of the family and we loved him very dearly. When he left to go back to his village a stronger, healthier, finer boy, he was better because of us and we were a lot better for having had him as our friend.

ELEVEN ·

THE WAR

Laos has been threatened by war ever since 1954 when she first established herself as a completely independent nation under the Geneva Agreement which followed the war in Indo-China. Sometimes in our village hospital high in the foothills of the Himalayas this threat of war seemed remote —the people were so gentle, the mountains were so impenetrable, the situation so apparently calm.

While I was in America in 1958 from January till June, Laos was run by a coalition government. An agreement had been reached at the end of 1957 by the two half-brothers, neutralist Prince Souvanna Phouma, then Prime Minister, and the Communist Prince Souphanouvong. Prince Souphanouvong's forces, the Pathet Lao, controlled the two large northeastern provinces, of Sam Neua and Phong Saly. He skillfully used his control of these two provinces as a lever to bargain his way into the royal government of Prince Souvanna Phouma. The neutralist Prince Souvanna Phouma did not seem to object, as long as the *status quo* were maintained. Many American, British and French advocates of Lao independence tried to point out to Souvanna Phouma the lessons of recent history, especially that of Czechoslovakia where only a few months after a "coalition" with Communists was completed, the nation fell. Nevertheless Prince Souvanna Phouma agreed to form a coalition government that included Communists.

Two Communist members, including Prince Souphanouvong, were given portfolios as Ministers, and 10 or 12 seats in the National Assembly were held by the Communist representatives of the two northeastern provinces. A plan was worked out to integrate the Pathet Lao army of 6,000 men into the Royal Lao army of 25,000 men. The Communist Pathet Lao force changed to a political party called the Neo Lao Hak Xat.

At this point, Prince Souvanna Phouma was replaced by a new Premier, Phoui Sananikone. He had been Premier for only a short time when I brought my team back to Laos in the summer of 1958. Sananikone had no confidence in the concept of a coalition government, when it was clearly the intention of part of the coalition to seize power at the earliest opportunity and remake Laos into a Communist country. In January, 1959, at his request the National Assembly scrapped the constitution. Then they voted the Premier special powers for a period of twelve months. Premier Sananikone then decided that the Pathet Lao soldiers who were still not integrated into the national army either had to be assimilated completely or disbanded. He also made matters extremely difficult for Communist politicians and kicked the two Communist leaders out of his Cabinet.

By July, 1959, it was obvious that the plan of integrating the Lao army was failing and that the Communist soldiers had no intentions of being assimilated into the national forces. They were being maintained as an independent Pathet Lao army by the Communist brass within the Royal Lao Army.

We first heard of the problem of army integration in June,

when the leader of the military battalion in Muong Sing called me over to the fortress to tell me that I was not to leave the village at night without an armed military escort. When I asked why, he said that the situation was becoming "*très grave.*" He told me that some Pathet Lao (Communist) troops south of us had forcibly resisted integration. When ordered to Luang Prabang, they had not obeyed, but deserted and fled into the mountains towards the borders of North (Communist) Viet Nam.

We had sporadic reports of war from our radio during the next few summer months. As usual the terrorist technique was monotonously familiar. Small, well-trained Communist bands would come out of hiding at midnight and attack a small isolated Lao army post or a house, killing, mauling and mutilating. Occasionally a story of atrocity and slow death would come to us. We listened to these reports and tried not to let them create fear, for fear is exactly the weapon that the Communists use in this whispering warfare of Laos.

The monsoon rains were pouring down and the sick were flooding into our hospital. We tried not to think about war. However, by the middle of the summer the distant rumblings became more like near thunder. Our Lao students were coming in late for work and often, when they did come, they were desperately exhausted. They had spent many hours the night before on patrol. During the daytime we would see the patrols marching out, and we would listen to their reports of the build-up of Communist forces on the China side of our northern frontier, five or six miles away.

The Lao army was doing an excellent job in eradicating internal jealousies among the soldiers. In each army battalion were Thai Dam, Thai Lu and others, as well as Lao themselves. The internal friction that existed between these tribes for centuries was being lessened by the new training programs which told the soldiers of their duties to their King, their nation and their flag. Our corpsmen came to our hospital filled with this new patriotism and new enthusiasm. We would hear them singing patriotic songs in the fort at night. Lao army training was progressing very well.

One afternoon out on a sick-call I came on a group of soldiers sitting in a field with their officer reciting on a melodic scale the fundamentals of the trigger-assembly of their rifle: "This is the trigger, this is the hammer, this is the head, and this is the screw," went their chant, just the way we sang our lessons as children.

The Lao are very touchy about their beliefs and superstitions relating to the origins of different tribes. Each tribe thinks itself superior to the others; the Lao group, for example, believe that their race is strongest. The legend about the origin of these races begins with a sacred pumpkin. An envoy of one of their ancient kings split this pumpkin up with a red hot poker. The first people to tumble out of the pumpkin were the aboriginal Kha, whose skin is a little dark because it was seared by the heat. Next came the lighter-colored mountain tribe of the Meo; finally came the lightest-skinned of them all, the Lao. There are anthropologists who take another view and believe that the people of Laos are simply the result of centuries of blending between the bloods of the Tibetan, the Burman, the Thai and the Yunanese.

What were the origins of the Communist group in Laos? They go back to 1953, during the Indo-China War, when the group was formed by Prince Souphanouvong, aided by Ho Chi Minh. They attacked Laos in 1953 and the armies of this force (the Pathet Lao) came perilously close to the capitol. In May, 1954, the war ended after the fall of the ill-fated fortress of Dien Bien Phu. Viet Nam was divided at the 17th parallel and in July, 1954, the United States Navy steamed into the harbor of Haiphong, to begin the historic evacuation of Vietnamese escapees from Communism.

That first day I looked upon the rocks of northern Indo-China, over five years ago, I wondered what this strange and mysterious area would be like. Now I was living in North Laos only a few hundred miles west, as the vulture flies, of my former refugee camps in Haiphong, centuries apart in some ways, and yet very close in the similarity of suffering.

The 1954 Geneva Agreement recognized the independence of Laos and its three million inhabitants. It also called for the withdrawal of all the Pathet Lao Communist fighting units into the provinces of Phong Saly and Sam Neua. The Geneva Treaty also provided for the withdrawal of the Viet Nam Communist forces. And there was established an International Control Commission composed of representatives of India, a neutral; Canada, a pro-Western; and Poland, a Communist nation. After the political settlement was signed by Prince Souphanouvong and Prince Souvanna Phouma in November, 1957, the two northern provinces were surrendered.

Early in 1958 the Lao government, under Premier Phoui Sananikone, stated that they believed that the unity of the nation was established, the armies were being integrated, and therefore the presence of the International Control Commission was no longer necessary. Any remaining problems should be dealt with by the elected government.

The political party called the Neo Lao Hak Xat, which is just another name for Communism, had become a strong internal threat. They had an organization that went right to the villages of Asia, whereas the other political parties, in the sudden sophistication of independence, sometimes did not reach deeply enough into the villages. How could they? These non-Communist parties had the arduous task of running the government, whereas the Neo Lao Hak Xat was free to criticize, condemn and poison.

On our river trips we would find the Neo Lao Hak Xat newspaper in every village along the river valley, and many young men and women trained to believe and accept the teachings of the Communists. Of course, they did not call themselves Communists, or advocate that they be made part of China. They spoke of the "terrible errors" of the Lao Royal Government and of the need for ox-carts instead of limousines. They constantly harped on the mistakes of Premier Sananikone's government, and the errors of American foreign aid. They magnified these out of all proportion.

My students loved to listen to our small transistor-run radio. There are two news broadcasts, one after lunch and one late in the evening. They would sit on the window sill, looking over into the sky of China, and hold the radio close against their ears. Earl once said to me, "There sits young Asia listening to her future."

On July 15, 1959, rebel attacks sharply increased in the two provinces of Sam Neua and Phong Saly. We heard that an emergency telegram was sent on July 24th asking the United States to supply experts to help train the army immediately in the use and maintenance of equipment.

Later in July the rebel guerillas attacked a 35-mile front in northeastern Sam Neua, not far from the famous fortress of Dien Bien Phu. Some radio reports said that as many as eight villages fell to the Communists. Others said there was heavy howitzer fire.

The people are a drowsy people, and the country is a landlocked country. It has been invaded repeatedly, but still it keeps its craggy individuality and the people fight courageously for their independence when they understand that it is threatened.

It seemed that it was threatened now. We often talked to our students about this threat to their nation. They understood that the Pathet Lao was simply an extension of the Communist Viet Minh movement, which in turn is an extension of Red China, which in turn is allied with Soviet Communism. They also seemed to understand that the simple fact that Premier Sananikone was making so much progress towards a strong, free nation had alarmed the Communists, who had decided to act immediately.

The Communists announced that the arrival of a 130-man American training mission for the Lao army was the cause of the blowup in August. They screamed on Radio Peking accusing the United States of "engineering" the Lao war and warning that the war in Laos could set all of Asia ablaze. Radio Peking and Radio Hanoi used language that was reminiscent of the Chinese intervention in Korea. The Chinese Communists called for an "abolition of all U. S. military bases" in Laos and warned that Washington must "bear full responsibility" for the Laos situation. In Hanoi the defense minister for the Communist leader Ho Chi Minh said that the fighting was a dangerous thing and Communist North Viet Nam would "not stand idly by."

The students understood that this propaganda was perfectly idiotic. They knew that no military bases were being built by the Americans, though certain former French bases were being improved in their physical setup by the Lao government forces. They were quick to distinguish lies from truth, and I think my young students were typical of all the young Laos. We tell them the truth, and their intelligence does the rest.

It is known that a considerable number of Pathet Lao were

taken into North Viet Nam, armed by North Vietnamese (Viet Minh) guns and formed into battalions. They were trained in the newer, more insidious techniques of the whispering war—the psychological battles. Their own rank and file were stiffened with Viet Minh hard-core Communist leaders. Now these troops were being sent back across the Lao border into their own land, to begin guerilla war against the Lao government. Their ways were devious: a midnight raid where only the village chieftain is slaughtered; an ambush killing a patrol of six men—never a large classical battle. Yet no one will ever prove that there was any "outside" intervention. Little did I realize that the United Nations itself would soon be involved in trying to prove who was fighting whom. My men were quick to see that indeed this was the same picture as the Communists' conquests elsewhere throughout the world.

By the month of August all of the land was ablaze with the news of the war. Airplanes came into the valley only rarely. The pilots told us that all planes had been requisitioned by the military, and no civilian regular runs were being made. "Four weeks and no mail plane yet; kind of tough on a guy with a six-months-old baby at home," commented Earl. Dwight, a little more staid, just said, "It sure gets lonesome without that airplane." I could only think of the danger. Should I consider taking my outfit out of a war-threatened area? Certainly, if war broke out along the Vietnamese frontier just a little east of us. China, close on our northern side, will be looking for provocative instances. Would they consider our hospital a provocation?

The Communist radio announcements became more and more arrogant. They brandished threats and accused us Americans in Muong Sing, while busily passing out cough medicine, of setting up spy stations and planning programs for eventual take-over of all of North Laos. Earl, Dwight and I smiled at each other. "We don't even entirely run our own hospital, so much of the work is done by our Lao student staff. So how are we possibly going to run North Laos?"

Every morning I would go across the muddy road (the monsoon turns the whole valley into a sea of mud) and speak to the Commandant. He was a bright young man, fast-talking and quick-thinking. I enjoyed being with him, and he did give me a good deal of information when I asked for it. But I always had to ask or, rather, wring it out of him. We listened to our radio, read the papers that came to us monthly, and blended this with the information from the Commandant.

The figures were staggering—1,500 men, 2,000 men, 15,000 men—invading Laos from Communist North Viet Nam. It seemed unreal that people were dying again in war. We knew that aggression, if expanded, could easily get out of hand. And we realized most of all that the tiny Kingdom of Laos, and the valleys just over our mountainside, possessed the potential for a catastrophe whose consequences might well alter the history of the world.

These things gave us many sleepless night. Was their goal war, or just unrest? To foment small local uprisings would keep the Lao government tremendously concerned in the expense and preparation of war. Perhaps this was part of the "initiate confusion within the Kingdom" program. The Communist government had attempted, by parliamentary means, to win over Laos but due to the bravery and strength of Premier Phoui Sananikone, they had failed. Now they were attempting to discredit western military help, western political aid, and especially American Economic Aid. Would they succeed?

One night while I was making a tape-recording, machine-gun fire broke out in the field across from my house. The whole sky was lit up with torches. My heart flipped, goose-flesh popped out all over, and I ran to the front porch of our house thinking, "They are attacking our village." The boys jumped out of bed and we looked quickly at the sky, alive with flares. The ratatatat of machine-gun fire was deafening.

We noticed that flares were falling right over the fortress. The sky was lit up with the blinding white brilliance of day. Another flare shot up from within the fortress. On looking closer, with cooler heads, we noticed that the machine-gun firing was coming from within the fortress. A few minutes later one of our student soldiers quietly ambled over to the hospital. We asked him, "Tao Souk, what are they doing? What is happening? Are they attacking Muong Sing?" Tao Souk looked at us, smiled at the perturbed Americans and said, "Oh, no, we just received a new shipment of ammunition by paradrop. You know, 50 per cent of the ammunition that we get is no good. We are just trying it out to see that it works."

I thought to myself, "What an alarmist you are, Dooley! Who's scared around here?" Nevertheless that night seemed a preview of the nights of horror that we feared would come. The local Commandant especially alarmed us when he told us that there was definite proof now of a build-up of Chinese troops on the Yunan border six miles north of us. It seemed as though they were going to push east from this border into Phong Saly at the same time that they were pushing west from North Viet Nam.

Few supply planes came in. I flew down to Vientiane on an airplane that came in the month of August, to have a long visit with Colonel Oudone Sananikone. Colonel Sananikone was a nephew of the Premier and belonged to one of the most capable and famous families of Laos. Colonel Oudone's wife was leader of the activities of the Lao women, and he was the Minister of Public Welfare and Health. This made him my boss, and an excellent boss he was. He gave me a free hand in the running of my hospital, yet he seemed to know every aspect of administration involved. He had visited my hospital twice in the past. As a Colonel, he was the most interested in our army training program. He was pleased that I did not make my hospital into a white man's hospital with a few Asian assistants, but rather an Asian hospital with three Americans working in it.

Colonel Oudone was a young man, about 34, stocky, and a veteran of many years of fighting. He was well-known through his land not only as a fighter, but as a thinker. Though not a heavy-set man, as are most of the Lao, he had extremely broad shoulders and a chin that jutted forward in almost arrogant fashion. His eyes were wide set and he had a heavy shank of hair over which his military cap perched straight and proper. Along with many other young Lao such as Sisouk Na Champassak, Impeng Suryadhay, Keo Viphathong, and others the Colonel made up the powerful political group called the C.D.I.N. which stand for Comité pour la Defense des Intêrets Nationaux, or Committee for the Defense of National Interests. These young men hold the future of the Kingdom in their capable hands. These men are dynamic and have a surging vitality. They also have a deep and profound love of their country, and are determined to serve it with loyalty. Upon attaining some power in the Phoui Sananikone government early in 1958 they attacked the corruption that had taken hold of the nation. They helped to abolish the former sloth and old corruption. They established rural self-help programs, village school programs, civic action programs, and made it their task to see that the young people became aware of their duties as citizens of the Kingdom of Laos.

A youth rally had been held in Vientiane and when Colonel Sananikone told me about this his eyes gleamed with pride. The youth rally had been set up by the Minister of Youth, Sisouk Na Champassak. Sisouk had formerly been in New York with the UN and I knew him well. The rally was the first of its kind, an old-fashioned rally, boy scout-jamboree and political convention combined. Thousands of students marched in parades through the city and out to a temple ground area several miles outside the capitol. Here they had an encampment, sang songs, made a huge bonfire, and listened to many talks. Colonel Sananikone told me how dynamic the young people were at this rally, and how anxious they were to improve themselves and their parents. They know now that there are better things in the world than they have yet achieved within their kingdom and they are determined to have them. In this same kind of search some have turned to Communism as the quicker way, forgetting that they must give up freedom they will never regain. With leaders like Sisouk, Colonel Sananikone, Impeng and Keo, the young people of the nation will be guided correctly. And I believe they will achieve what they seek. But I believe they need more assurance of the fact that the young men of the Western World will also respond to their challenge. They need our hands, our hearts, our economic support, and our diplomatic prestige.

Colonel Sananikone told me that at present they were not evacuating any wounded to the hospital at Muong Sing. They felt that this would be simply increasing the danger in the area, taking wounded men from one war zone and moving them into another threatened zone. He did, however, ask me to keep my hospital alerted for emergencies, and increase our training program to make more corpsmen capable of handling battle casualties. I pledged that we would.

He also told me of a program that had been in effect for several months wherein the Lao military groups around the country were trying to win the villages over to their side. I had seen evidence of this under the civilian program headed by Colonel Sananikone called Civic Action. The Colonel pointed out that there was also a Military Civic Action program whereby the military would aid the people of various villages. He said that this was tremendously important in the two provinces where the war was going on. I left the Colonel pleased and proud to be working hand in hand with a government such as his.

Premier Phoui Sananikone invited me to a small stag dinner in his home, which was his way of saying, "God bless, and we're glad to have you here, Dooley." There was a lot of friendly give-and-take at this dinner, and although politics were not discussed and very little was said about the war, I returned to Muong Sing feeling that the capital was fully aware of the danger of Laos being pushed into war deeper and deeper.

A few days later I loaded another plane with supplies, and returned to my village. I was reassured of the Lao government's support and interest in my mission, though I was apprehensive about the turn for the worse that the war was taking.

(*Postscript in 1960.* As this book goes to press in the early months of 1960, the political situation in Laos has changed from what it was during the period covered above. Late in 1959 Premier Phoui Sananikone reversed his anti-Communist stance in favor of "neutralism." Seven members of his Cabinet resigned and the C.D.I.N. demanded that a provisional government be established. The Prime Minister thereupon handed in his resignation to King Savang Vatthana. A new Cabinet headed by Kou Abhay as Premier, and his brother, Nhouy, as Vice Premier, became the compromise administration and restored civil authority after a week of army rule. Dag Hammarskjold, Secretary-General of the UN, had wired the King: "I permit myself to express the hope that the line of independent neutrality . . . will be firmly maintained." *Time* reported the news of the civilian compromise Cabinet by saying, "It was, everyone in Vientiane delightedly agreed, a truly Lao solution: though Premier Phoui Sananikone had been ousted, his new, more neutralist policy, at least for the time being, had won." The Abhay interim government is to rule until the national elections scheduled for April, 1960.)

TWELVE • A SHEET OF BLUE PAPER

Now we spent every noon listening to the radio news. Occasionally we listened to the Voice of America. More often we heard British news stations better. In the evenings we listened to Communist Radio Hanoi, realizing that, though most of what they said were macabre lies, they revealed their aims and tactics "between the lines." We learned that the Communists had attacked several villages in the area of Phong Saly, though the radio broadcast said they were now retreating. The Royal Lao Army dropped parachutists between Communist rebel troops and their Viet Minh headquarters, thus cutting off their supply line. The guns captured during this maneuver were made in Communist Czechoslovakia. Everyone in this area knew these facts but they also knew that, in the event of the United Nations being brought into the matter, further more definite proof would probably be demanded.

Many people in Muong Sing were speaking of the fact that the Lao government had sent airplanes to Sam Neua to evacuate families of the Lao government employees. I considered this bad news. Seemingly the Lao government was abandoning Sam Neua and letting the Communist come. On the night of August 5 the war news was very bleak indeed. The Lao government put all northern provinces on an "alert."

My boys and I had put our hospital on an alert also and began war-training exercises. The next morning we started teaching all of the students how war wounded should be brought in. We discussed the unloading of wounded from an airplane, and decided how stretchers should be put on our jeep. We taught the men how to open and carry stretchers and how to make additional emergency stretchers from bamboo and blankets. We practiced such emergency measures as admitting 15, 20, and 25 patients into the wards at one time. We showed the students how the patients should be stripped, their clothes put under their heads, and their bodies covered with blankets. We discussed how they would be tagged on the foot and how morphine when given would be marked on the forehead. We held classes on first-aid and on triage. In essence we began a long course of training our men for emergency work.

The boys and I discussed what we would do in a dangerous emergency ourselves. Would we evacuate and abandon our hospital? We were told that the Filipinos of Operation Brotherhood were forced to leave their village hospital in the war-plagued province of Sam Neua. Operation Brotherhood is that grand program of the Filipinos, who have several medical teams scattered throughout Laos—they are doing a topnotch job. They give of themselves. Now the problem must be considered: if I were ordered out by the Lao or the American Ambassador, should I go, or should I refuse the order? And if I went should I take all my civilian crew with me?

Abandoning my hospital would be difficult. If I thought this hospital were to be destroyed, it would be doubly difficult. It would be destroying part of me. I did not think the

Communists could be that stupid; a hospital is above politics. It can serve humanity, no matter what the political coloring of this humanity.

It would be a difficult thing for me to take myself out of the geographical position that demanded the presence of a doctor. I had been under threat for many years. I had lived under the ogre of Communist conquest, and I had seen Communism at close hand. I was not afraid of this any more. There had been a time when I was; now I was not. I am a doctor, I am supposed to take care of people who are sick, especially the wounded. The root, the foundation, the heart of it all was that I am a doctor.

At one point Chai said, "Doctor, you go. You are American, the war is a Lao war." But Ngoan said, "Deep down in my heart I know that you will stick by us Lao." I too knew that we would stick by them.

I had seen what Communists do to Asians who work with Americans, for I had Asians working with me in North Viet Nam when the Communists took over. I knew that the six or eight of my star pupils would be taken out and beheaded in front of the whole village and their heads, with the organs of the neck hanging down, would be impaled upon stakes. I knew that the Communists would take members of my Lao crew, stand them in a circle facing inward, and with machetes would deftly cut the tendons in the back of their knees. When the crew would fall to the ground the Communists would walk around and hack them to pieces. I have seen the Communists do this and just leave the men in the middle of a room or in a field. When the tendons were cut, the Lao would not bleed to death. They would crawl like animals until they were caught and hacked to death. This is what they would do to Chai, to Si, to Ngoan, and to Deng. To the girls on my staff they would do even more dreadful things. These were the thoughts that burned the hours of my nights those early weeks of August. The decision was mine and only mine.

This is a time when we must be strong and courageous, even though fear might spread through our bones. The first week of August was even more difficult than usual because I was alone. I had sent Earl to Vientiane for supplies and Dwight was in Cambodia with our team there for a few days.

I wanted to indicate to my Lao students that I had confidence in them. I wanted to show them that I knew they could maintain and sustain me and my hospital when my two Americans were gone. And indeed they did. They bent over backwards helping each other and helping me, though they often spun their wheels just a little bit. They stepped on each other and on me; the operating-room was often so crowded that we continuously contaminated each other. Ngoan gave all of the anesthesia for me and the Lao scrubbed as surgical nurses. It pleased me to see how well they did these things.

Perhaps I felt a great deal more loneliness at this time because I had no one with whom to speak English. I frequently found myself looking in the mirror and saying, "Hello, Tom. My, you look fine today."

I had some difficulty with the Military Commandant while Earl and Dwight were gone. He wanted to take Deng and others, my finest crew, and transfer them down into the central portion of the province. Of all times I needed a trained crew more than ever at this moment. I had to argue with all my force to prove my point. I won it, but it was a constant irritation to both of us, to say nothing of the amount of effort required not to get something accomplished but merely preserved.

Very late in the afternoon of August 6th, a plane circled overhead. It was the first plane we had seen for several weeks. We went to the airfield to find Earl disembarking. Earl had left from Vientiane, but due to the war had been held up in Luang Prabang for several days. Finally he went to the Commandant of the Lao army in Luang Prabang and explained his predicament and they turned an airplane over to him. All military as well as civilian planes had been requisitioned for evacuation of civilians from the war-torn areas around Sam Neua. However the Commandant helped out and flew Earl back to us.

Earl was full of news of the war, and of the things that were happening in the capital, and I hungered for accuracy. It was strange that the only way we heard of the war was through rumors and the radio. That was the most deadly factor of the struggle—it was never black or white, always a nebulous gray.

After the Lao students greeted Earl and heard all the news from the capital, Earl said he would like to have a few minutes with me in private. The dark sincerity that came across his face frightened me. When we were alone, he pulled out a letter given to him by the American Ambassador to Laos, Mr. Horace Smith.

The letter was dated August 3rd and began: "Dear Tom, The Royal Government has reported many insurgent attacks on border posts in Sam Neua and considerable penetration into the Phong Saly from the east. Most of these attacks appear to involve incursions from across the border." I read that paragraph without alarm because we had heard this news of Phong Saly, a neighboring province of ours. The letter went on to point out that there were reports of recent Red Chinese troop movements, involving some three hundred to four hundred people, on our border some five miles away. We had also heard the same thing, although our figures were double.

The Ambassador wrote that "from information so far available, the American Embassy fears that the Royal Army may be unable to guarantee your continued security and, as you know, the Embassy is not in a position to guarantee that you or your assistants will have an opportunity to evacuate safely if the situation develops rapidly.

"I therefore urge you to consider carefully the desirability of either evacuating immediately your assistants and yourself at least temporarily, to a place of safety such as Luang Prabang or Vientiane until the situation is clarified, or of making arrangements that satisfy you that you will be able to do so whenever it becomes necessary."

This was it! A letter from the American Ambassador—not ordering me, for he knew he could not—yet "urging" that I consider the desirability of leaving—*now*. This was exactly what I had given so much thought to. This was the first step in a program that might end up in tragedy. I had already decided that I would not evacuate and this letter did not change my feeling. I had also sent a telegram to the Commandant of the First Military Region of the Lao Army, informing him that our hospital was ready and able to receive any war wounded that he wished to send here.

I then wrote a letter to the Ambassador, knowing it might not get out for many weeks. I informed him that I appreciated his letter and his consideration, but felt that my duty was here in the hospital. I wrote: "We are not going to evacuate at this time. From my rapport with the Royal Army both locally and at staff level, I am confident that if the situation warrants they will do all in their power to give us security and, if necessary, evacuation.

"I have requested the army to consider our hospital as

a Lao military hospital. Further I have asked that we be evacuated only when and if it becomes necessary to evacuate the military units of this area. At such time I shall request first priority and am sure all possible aid will be given to us."

I went on to point out to the Ambassador that if the local civilian authorities ordered us to evacuate, I would turn the decision over to the Royal Army. If there were sick and wounded in Muong Sing, then it was our duty to stay with them. Above all else it must be remembered that we are a medical unit. I also said, "However, if ordered by the Lao Military we shall evacuate immediately."

I have great admiration for Ambassador Smith and I tried to explain fully my feeling: "I feel very strongly, sir, that we three Americans are now given a splendid opportunity to serve our nation and the Kingdom of Laos. By being present in this village at their time of need, by not seeking self-safety, we can reaffirm (in a minute way) America's policy: when free people are threatened, when Taiwans, Laos and Lebanons are intimidated, America will stand by their people and not abandon them." I wrote the letter and felt relieved that my decision had been reached and announced. I told Earl what I had done—he was 100 per cent in accord. We both wished that Dwight were with us now. We knew that when he heard the news of the increase in the war, he would come home immediately, though we also knew he would have the same difficulty that Earl had with transportation. There was strength in all three of us together.

The Lao Army now began an intense recruiting program in our area. In one week we had over 100 admission physical exams to do for them. Every day there were drills and marches on the fields beside our house. Every afternoon there was shooting out on the rifle-range. The whole village was alarmed. Early in the morning of August 8 we received a police radio message that Dwight was stranded in Nam Tha. His small plane was forced down by the rains.

The telegram came while we were eating breakfast but almost simultaneously, through the dawn's mist, we heard the motor of an airplane. We knew it must be Dwight so we raced out to the airport, as fast as we could in knee-deep mud. We watched the plane cut down through the mist and land in one of the worst landings that I had ever seen. Why the wheels weren't fractured off, I do not understand. Dwight shakily came off the plane along with Dr. John Keshishian, the head of the MEDICO team in Viet Nam, who was here for a visit of several days. With them was our good friend, Bob Burns, the "typist in the army of the Lord."

They told me how their plane had taken off the day before and flown a terrible flight. They had circled Muong Sing, but could not land due to the fog. Instead they had gone to Nam Tha to land. Earlier this morning their plane had taxied to the end of the grass runway at Nam Tha to take off, but the wheels had sunk into the mud. The villagers at Nam Tha had grabbed the wheels and with the help of a jeep had managed to get the plane out of the mud. All baggage and passengers except Dwight and Doctor Keshishian had to get off to lighten the plane. The villagers laid a few extra bamboo mats, the pilot gunned the plane, released the brakes, and catapulted into the air, taking off almost vertically.

Dwight quietly said, "Worst flight I ever had." The French pilot was much more eloquent. "Twenty years I fly in Asia, always in these dangerous territories—never, never have I been as frightened as today." He added, "And for two Americans."

I quizzed the pilot about the war. He told me that the landing strips at Phong Saly and Sam Neua were under attack and were jammed with civilians and military refugees, waiting for a plane to evacuate them. There was no order or discipline whatever, people were all over the landing strip clogging and blocking it. Disorder and confusion reigned, the familiar chaos of Asian war.

The pilot told us that he saw one village landing strip where many people had been beheaded. Their heads were stuck up on posts along the side of the strip. As the plane came to land, the pilot spotted this atrocity, pulled back on the stick and flew away. The Communists fired on his plane with small weapons. I asked a foolish question: "Were the victims military or not?" The pilot said simply, "I saw only the head and the vessels of the neck hanging down. I could not tell if they were military or not." We heard another figure, over 300 killed and several hundred more wounded.

Dr. Keshishian obviously had little idea what he was getting himself involved in. He had come up to visit us on his way home from working with our team in Viet Nam, and we were glad to have a surgeon at a time like this. Bob Burns was always a welcome visitor; though he probably would pass out at the sight of blood, we had plans for him.

At midnight that night Earl, Dwight, Bob and I discussed what I had decided. I knew my refusal to evacuate was right. I said: "Nothing is obscure, nothing is in a tangle." I knew exactly what I must do. No one in Vientiane, in New York, or anywhere else could judge the situation as well as I could. We were lucky to have this chance. We would not abandon these people; we would stay here as long as we were needed. Bob Burns said he would carry our letter back to the Ambassador and explain our feelings more completely.

He had come to sound us out thoroughly, for the Ambassador suspected I might refuse his "urging."

On the plane that brought Dwight and Dr. Keshishian we found a great deal of mail. It was full of clippings about the war in Laos, and we learned more from the clippings than we did from the government of the place where we were living. A great deal of the mail upset me this particular day. Ordinarily mail pleases me; when people write and say "God bless" or ask for my autograph, I am a typical Irishman and delighted. However, because of my frame of mind and the darkness all around us, on this day I was angry. Many months later I found a copy of the letter I had written to my mother in St. Louis on this night of August 8. What I said was not very pretty. This is what I wrote:

Don't people in America know I've got my own problems just living from day to day? I am not interested in how much people are going to pay when I come to America for my lecture tour. I am very honored that Mutual of Omaha Company has decided to give me their Criss Award. I am tremendously pleased that they are giving me $10,000 to help run my hospital. I have planned to return the end of October to receive this Award and to stay on for a month's lecture tour. But this is months away and right now I have no time to think about this. Right now I must battle from day to day and work out the problems of war, death and chaos. People write and ask me to write another book, and tell me how I must find words. Don't they realize I have other things to do now?

I am a doctor. This is the root of me—I am a doctor. Everything else, everyone, is second to that. First, I am a doctor. All my duties are entwined with that and they are clear and lucid. Everything else is second. Home life, social life, writing life, living life, loving life, family, friends, romance, fame, fortune, all these are secondary, because I am a doctor. Perhaps I take this too much to heart. It was a hard and humiliating fight for me to become a doctor. I want Ambassadors to stop thinking of me as an international figure and a threat to the tranquility of their post. I want publishers to stop thinking of me as a hand that holds a conversation with a typewriter, while a piece of paper listens in. I want broadcasting systems to stop thinking of me as a correspondent and stop sending me telegrams asking for my opinion of the news. I want the people who write to me simply asking for my autograph to stop writing. There is nothing I can do about certain Senators' views on the excellency of my mission. I do not care whether the American Economic Mission considers me annoyingly autonomous or not. I disapprove of some people getting me so cheaply as a "wonderful" speaker and writing me how proud they are of this fact. Perhaps I am ranting and raving, but this is how I feel.

It is very late, close to three in the morning, and everyone is asleep in the house, even the frogs and insects of the jungle seem quiet tonight. Through the screen doors I can see tonight's moon. It is a lurid moon looking down on grisly things. Hundreds of dead in the north, major villages fallen to the Reds, a build-up of troops only a few miles away from us. Young men and women beheaded with their heads stuck on posts at the runway. The whole of the north suffering, bleating and crying, full of sadness. No wonder everything is quiet tonight. They are sad, soundlessly.

The letter stopped at this point and started again on Sunday, August 9, as follows:

The dawn came today wild and fiery. There was a turbulence of cloud and wind and rain. And then almost miraculously (and I expect miracles here all the time) the thunder stopped and the lightning no longer staggered across the sky and the whole valley fell into unearthly silence. We all noticed the noise of the silence. But then by noon the windless skies again grew disturbed and the sound of thunder was distant. Or was it the sound of guns? We never know now. The noise rolled and crashed overhead, and the skies streaked with lightning and opened up and once again flooded our valley. Dr. Keshishian is overwhelmed by the rains. The visiting Bob Burns is amazed at the downpour. I am scared. Scared.

I wrote letters like this, long letters to my friends all around the world, to my mother, knowing that it would take weeks and weeks before they would ever get these letters.

But by writing I talked to people just as though they were sitting across from me. How grateful I was to be able to talk, to write, to communicate.

In my village, we still experienced the madness of not-knowing; that same madness that had frightened the people into another exodus out of the neighboring provinces. We spent August 10, 11, and 12 working at the hospital training, doing physical examinations for the new army men. We made up emergency evacuation packs and planned the route. I talked into the tape-recorder, keeping a log of the day by day occurrences, never realizing to what use I would put this at a later date.

As I write these pages, going in spirit back across those monsoon months I remember very vividly the bizarre behavior of Earl and Dwight after Dwight's return from Cambodia. I remember certain incidents that took place in those early weeks of August—especially the boys' solicitousness. They knew I had been alone for a while so I assumed that was the reason why they were overly attentive to me. They poured my coffee, heated the water, ran the bulk of sick call. They told me, "Oh, let's not do that surgery today, doctor, you've already worked hard enough," whereas their usual comment was, "Oh, let's not quit, doctor; we have time to do one more operation."

The selection of food was made with great care during those evenings. Instead of just saying to Si, "Cook up another chicken," the boys were now saying, "Si, the doctor needs to gain a little weight, let's make some potatoes tonight." I vaguely noted these things at the time.

I also distinctly remember one late afternoon coming back from the hospital from surgery. Surgery is always tiring to me because of the intense concentration that it takes. I collapsed on the couch in the center room and one of my

Lao students came over and asked me if I wanted a back rub. I thought this was nice of her and said: "Why, of course, give the old man a back rub. But be careful of the scar on my side." I meant the scar where that little lump had been removed by Dr. Van Valin a few weeks before. The student nurse gave me a fine back rub and I did feel better. There was still some aching around the shoulder and the chest and some tenderness where the lump had been taken out. Their solicitousness was a warm and heartening thing. I did not realize what was behind it until much later.

Every afternoon we would listen to the news. Things seemed quiet and there was little change. Bob agreed with my letter to the Ambassador and said that he intended to take the next plane out when and if one ever came. At noon on Wednesday, August 12, just after we had scheduled surgery, we heard a small plane fly in. It was an old and tired Beechcraft belonging to the civilian Lao airline. Dr. Keshishian and Bob went to the airport, climbed aboard, and we said farewell.

This plane brought in some more mail; once again we were able to find out a little more about what was happening in areas so very close and so very threatening to us. On the night of August 11 I wrote in my notes: "The Voice of America announced today that over 4,000 Red troops were in the area of Sam Neua and Phong Saly, massing on the Vietnamese side of the frontier, a new attack was expected soon, or at the time of the end of the rains in October."

Four days later was Saturday, August 15. This was the day on which I read the blue sheet of paper—the telegram from Dr. Peter Comanduras, which I describe in the opening chapter of this book.

THIRTEEN ·

NOR EAR CAN HEAR, NOR TONGUE CAN TELL

Continuing the story from the point where I broke it off in Chapter One—that is, during my airplane flight west towards England—I arrived at London airport disheveled, crumpled and still depressed. I went to the Pan American window, where they immediately put me on a connecting flight to New York. On Thursday evening I arrived in New York, only a couple of days after leaving Muong Sing.

As I walked through Customs at International Airport, I looked up at the huge glass window and saw Dr. Peter Comanduras waiting for me. How good it was to see him! That night Peter, Gloria Sassano and I, the original three who had started MEDICO a short nineteen months previously, talked of many things. It was strange that in talking to them about myself I felt as though I were discussing the sickness of another person, not myself at all.

It was good to have Peter with me because he spoke to me not only as a doctor but as a father and a friend. He said, "The diagnosis has been confirmed with the National Institute of Health. It is malignant melanoma in the metastatic stage." I knew melanoma to be one of the most rapid-growing and most insidious kinds of tumors. I had malignant melanoma and in its metastatic state it already involved the lymph nodes under my arm. It was one of these nodes, the lowest one along the upper chest wall, that Doctor Van Valin had excised that afternoon in Muong Sing. Peter questioned me as a doctor, asking me whether or not I had a cough; I knew he was concerned about a spread of the cancer to my lung. He asked me if I had any soreness in the bones of my chest, fearing the cancer might have invaded the bone structure of my thorax.

Now I understood why I was having all the discomfort and weight loss over the past several months. I kept associating this with the fall on the river trip. This was not the cause though it certainly might have been an aggravation.

That first long night in New York was also made a lot easier by my brother, Malcolm. He flew in from Detroit that night and we talked of the weeks ahead. He was a great help, a sheltering tree, and I thank God for such a brother.

Malcolm and Peter both agreed that I would have to notify my mother immediately. But how? If I just said, "I have cancer," it would be a terrible shock to her. She had had so many shocks, having lost two husbands and two children. I first called a friend of ours in Saint Louis and asked her to go to my mother's and make sure that she would be all right when my call came. Malcolm and I planned how I would phrase this, and very carefully I called: "Hello, Mother. This is Tom. I am in New York. Yes, I'm all right but I have come home because I have to have some surgery done."

She immediately poured out questions. At first she was so relieved that I was no longer in North Laos that I thought she was having some kind of mental block. I said, "Mother, are you all right? Do you understand me? I am in New York."

"Yes, son. I know you are in New York and I'm so glad. I was so afraid you would be taken prisoner and tortured by the Communists. The war news has been so terrible. I worry about you and I sleep so little."

She sounded relieved and I knew I had to say then that I had cancer. "Mother, I have just discovered that I have a tumor which is believed to be malignant. Do you understand me, Mother?"

"Yes, I understand, dear. You have a tumor that may be malignant. Well, you take good care of yourself, dear."

I knew that I had still not broken through the fog of the initial shock. Later my mother told me that it wasn't until the next day, when she actually saw it in the newspaper, that she fully realized how serious was the cause of my returning to America.

Malcolm left and the following day I flew home to Saint Louis. I had to see my mother and explain to her in person the truth of the cancer that I faced. Mother met me at the airport and soon I was home again. From her strength I was able to derive much. She had been through a great deal of unhappiness in her life, and had a staunch way of taking all this though I knew it was so terrible for her. At Mass the next morning, in the same Cathedral that I had attended as a child, I prayed to the same God to Whom I had prayed all around the world. I had some peace but little solace.

That same night I flew back to New York and the following morning entered Memorial Hospital. Peter sent me to the world-famous pathologist Dr. George Papanicolaou who in turn took me to the country's great specialist in this kind of cancer-surgery, Dr. Gordon McNeer. He made all the arrangements for me to enter this hospital.

I tried to feel that I was prepared for what was ahead, but one is never completely prepared. Everything was strange. Instead of the familiar feelings that I have when walking into a hospital, things now seemed new and I felt apprehensive. The hospital had the usual odor of ether and sterile solutions, well known to me, but today it was strangely peculiar. The hospital bed seemed much different now that I was in it, instead of standing over it speaking to a patient.

From the barrage of tests, needles, x-rays and examinations I knew that my doctors were probing around my body, digging deep into its recesses for evidence of extension of my cancer. The final decision as to how radical the surgery would be depended upon how deep the involvement was. If it extended into my neck and arm nodes, the operation might include amputation of my right arm at the shoulder. With one arm I could do little in Laos.

On my third day my doctor came into my room and said, "Tom, all tests have proven negative for extension of the cancer. It seems that the melanoma involves only the chest wall and the local lymph nodes. Tomorrow we will do an extensive removal of all the skin muscles, nodes, veins, nerves and tissue of the right side of your chest and axilla. We can graft skin from your legs to put on the bare chest wall. We'll operate tomorrow."

In spite of the weeks of pain that I knew would be ahead, I felt good. Maybe things would come out all right. I offered up a little prayer of thanks and said, "All right, Doctor, I'm ready." He grinned and said, "Good. Chin up, boy."

All the familiar preparations began, things that so many times in the past I had ordered for other patients. Now it was my turn for the presurgical bath, the premedications the night before, the shaving of axilla and all the chest wall. And then a very heavy night sleep, well drugged from premedication seconal.

The following morning the priest came early to bring me

Holy Communion. I wondered then, as I so often do, how do people live without their faith? In whose hands can they put their troubled selves and the infinity of questions that come to a man at a time like this? After Holy Communion, I had a few moments of thanksgiving and felt serener, safer, stronger. I was in His hands now, wholly, and in resignation. Peace of soul and body flooded over me, a deep, warm, quiet peace. I was ready.

A few hours later they came in to give me my premedication hypo. I was scheduled for surgery after high noon. I smiled to myself and thought about "high noon" back in my valley in Muong Sing. I knew the medication was working, but fear was also gnawing deeply into me. A normal reaction, I knew, but this knowledge lessened the fear's intensity not one iota.

The man in the green operating-room gown rolled my nearly drugged body off my bed onto the hard stretcher and I was wheeled up to the operating-room. I felt sure that they had given me more than the usual dose. Sure is tough to quiet Dooley down. As we wheeled into the operating-room I remember noticing a lot of people standing around the room who seemed uncomfortable in their masks and gowns and caps. They were part of a television crew that was going to photograph the operation. Then my arm was strapped to the arm board and the anesthetist very gently put the needle in. I knew this would be sodium pentathol. As the drug was injected in my veins, two strong hands came over my eyelids and pushed them down shut. I remember nothing else, nothing else.

A day and a half later (I'm told) I had lucid moments. I remember waking up for a few minutes, looking around the recovery room, everything spinning around again and blurring, and then to sleep. A few hours later, or was it minutes, or was it days, I woke up once again. I remember very distinctly a recovery nurse, who had a heavy German accent. I was angry at her, because she wouldn't let me fling myself around the bed the way I wanted to. I remember cussing at her in German.

I remember seeing Dr. Peter Comanduras looking down over me in the recovery room. His cool mien gave me reassurance, even in the haze of anesthesia. Later when I was wheeled to my room I remember seeing mother, and her warm love gave me much confidence. Then came the slow recovering of consciousness, of focusing on objects in the room. I remember the tightness in my chest and the raw soreness in my legs. I knew that there were normal postoperative pains.

I was determined to take no morphine shots for pain. I was operated on Thursday, the 27th of August, less than a week after I left Laos. By Saturday the 30th I was wide awake, sitting up in bed, sore as hell all over.

On Sunday I had some visitors and a bourbon on the rocks. I felt much better now. By Monday they let me out of bed to walk around a little bit, though I walked around all bent over like an old man. Later, Gloria Sassano came over to the hospital, bringing several baskets of mail from the office of MEDICO. How the mail was pouring in and how wonderful the letters were from all around the world, wishing me good luck, and the blessing of God.

It seemed the newspapers were carrying every single development of Dooley's illness. I had had no idea what a personal shock my cancer was to so many people around the world. A lady in Ecuador wrote that she was praying for me; a litany was being offered by Carmelite nuns in Fort Worth, Texas; Hindu prayers were offered for me near Delhi where someone was sitting crosslegged on the floor, reading the *Bhagavad-Gita.* I knew that the public in America was interested in my work, but I was overwhelmed that my sickness would cause such reaction. For many years I have received as many as two and three thousand letters a month, but now I was receiving several thousand letters a day. The spiritual bouquets that were offered up for Dooley must have perfumed the halls of heaven. I felt their strength and knew their power.

I received many strange letters from well-meaning people. They kept me gratified though sometimes amused. One lady suggested that I check on the new research in vitamins and thyroid relationships, and a letter came from the University of Munich suggesting some animal gland injection. An Anglican bishop on the West Coast told me that he would pray for me "from time to time." A lady 77 years old suggested that I rub burnt alum on my chest, as this would make my cancer go away. Another wonderful lady suggested that I eat alfalfa and garlic, pointing out to me that quinine and digitalis were acquired from these sources by the early South American Indians. She told me that alfalfa contained every vitamin so far discovered, as well as ten of the eleven mineral elements. My dear correspondent also pointed out that although alfalfa lacks in carbohydrates I could supply that by eating potatoes, "But always raw, never cooked."

One man wrote and told me "if it is any consolation to know that you have scores of friends you have met who are deeply concerned for your welfare, then you should be much consoled. I am an elevator operator and in the course of my day I overhear, without eavesdropping, many conversations. You are the topic under discussion many, many times. I doubt that you know any of the people who work in this building. I certainly do not, but they all know of you and your work and your sickness to them was a personal blow."

What a wonderful way to learn that people are rooting for you—on elevators.

Another woman wrote and said: "I do not know whether you have ever heard of the urine therapy. Probably not. It is far too simple for the medical profession as a whole to give credence to it. But since you are in the category far above the rank and file I hope you will see the wisdom of checking into this. I suggest you buy the book entitled *The Water of Life.*" The spirit in which the letter was written was wonderful, though I was not quite ready to try her therapy.

A man in Joshua, Texas, had a particular weed concoction he wanted to send to me because he believed that it would help. The children of my favorite Texan family, the Womacks of Fort Worth, composed new words to the tune of "Hang Down Your Head, Tom Dooley," and they sent them on to me:

Lift up your heart, Tom Dooley,
Your work will never die.
You taught us to love our neighbor
And not just to pass him by.

We'll pray for you, Tom Dooley,
Your cure and your patients, too.
We'll send in our dimes and dollars
For work that's left to do.

Lift up your head, Tom Dooley,
Lift up your head, don't cry.
Lift up your head, Tom Dooley,
'Cause you ain't a-goin to die.

One lady just wrote a letter to my office, and said, "Here's another why for which there is no human answer. Did God raise Tom Dooley up, give him a certain fire to blaze a trail in the wilderness, to give his brilliant mind and healing hands to the lost and ignorant and diseased? Did God bring Tom Dooley up to leave his stamp of greatness on each person with whom he comes in contact that are never quite the same again and then perhaps recall him from this world, his mission fulfilled, and MEDICO his memorial?" I wondered to myself if this was what the Lord had intended. But I did not think so.

Another lady wrote and said, "It's too bad that his life so dedicated now is in mortal danger. His beloved Laos is besieged. It seems that both are besieged." Another said, "One moment I faced agonizing death. The next moment I face God, and now I have a new release." She said that I should get in contact with a man named Oral Roberts. She added a postscript and said, "You are too valuable and lots of happiness lays ahead of you, see Oral Roberts, be cured, be cured." Someone else wrote me enclosing a long mimeographed article entitled "My Operation." Nice light reading for a convalescent!

I received letters from Columbia, South America, Ecuador, Poland, India, Australia. A lady from France suggested yogurt, black bread, no sugar, soy beans, and Vitamin E in large dosages. (Doesn't she know that Vitamin E is a sexual stimulant?)

Another man wrote: "My dear Doctor, Be of good courage. Cancer is caused by eating flesh foods. It can be healed by prayer. Do not fear cancer. You do not need surgery. Just pray." He signed it and then said, "I invite comments." Somehow or other the surgical staff of the Memorial Hospital does not completely agree with him, though we all give faith a lot of credit.

One of the most touching gifts I received was a scroll from a small village in Korea. On the scroll were written the Beatitudes in Korean, and with it the wish that my health would soon improve and that I would return to the people of Asia.

Another woman took a more aggressive attitude. She said, "Go ahead, throw your life away, but don't feel sorry for yourself. I and your friends feel bad enough about your troubles." Another woman sent me a lovely Biblical quotation which said, "Here, at whatever hour you come, you will find light, health and happiness, human kindness." I thought to myself if I ever write a book about this problem I am going to call it "at whatever hour you come." I will, the next one I write.

Another cheery card came from the bartender of a small bar I used to go to in St. Louis, called "Petit Pigalle." Some children wrote me and said they hoped my "lump glands" were not involved. I think they meant "lymph" but lump is more descriptive.

One lady wrote me and said, "I'm sending you my secret for good health. All you have to do is this (and keep it quiet). Keep all dishes boiled, never eat food that you or anyone else have handled unless the food is thoroughly cooked; and, above all things, do not eat out of aluminum pans." Evidently she has no friends at Alcoa.

A lady from Kankakee (through which I had traveled many a day when a student at Notre Dame) said, "Today I am sending you a miracle healing from my hands. By touching this paper and the writing of this pen the cancer will be burned out of your body. Now you are full of pep and vigor again. Do not doubt me or you will not get it."

I thank all these people who wrote. I thank them for the thought that was at hand. However foolish the suggestion seemed, however unrealistic the advice, the kind intention and the depth of spirit are what count.

One night I dreamed that I was walking up a steep trail, leading across my valley floor and weaving its way through the high rain forest onto the mountain top just east of us. My boys were with me, and some of my Lao students. And in the vivid flash of the moment, in my dream, I saw a century-old pagoda that nestles on this mountain slope. The pagoda is made of mud stones and is crowned by a high spire. Hanging from the spire are long white banners, the streamers of Buddhist prayers. There are miniature bells that tinkled in the wind.

I have often been there before. But in the dream I reconstructed it even more lucidly. The central stupa has a shrine below it. Black and silver images and cascades of bells, big and small, fall down from the slope of the stupa. As I looked around through the eyes of my dream I saw many areas of land around this mountain slope, where the jungle had been burned and the mountain's naked ground was dull black. I also saw tiny insignificant little figures of men on these patches of brown earth. These men were planting the new rice seedlings into the burnt soil. The month of my dream must have been May, the time of lilacs at my beloved Notre Dame. But in Laos, May is a time when the season is driest. These are the nights that they burn the mountain.

The mountain in my dream was burned, and now they were planting the new life into the near dead soil. I dreamed this clearly and when the blue turquoise of morning came, though perhaps neither ear could hear nor tongue could tell, I knew the meaning of my dream.

From my hospital bed in New York, with the same white light of revelation I had known once several years before, I saw what I must do. After Communion that morning, Tuesday, the first of September, my God and my dream commanded me. I must, into the burnt soil of my personal mountain of sadness, plant the new seedlings of my life—I must continue to live. I must cultivate my fields of food, to feed those who cannot feed themselves.

The concept came to me as strongly and as powerfully as if a peal of bronze bells proclaimed it. There was no more self-sadness, no darkness deep inside: no gritty annoyance at anyone or anything. No anger at God for my cancer, no hostility to anyone. I was out of the fog of confusion—standing under the clear light of duty.

The jagged, ugly cancer scar went no deeper than my flesh. There was no cancer in my spirit. The Lord saw to that. I would keep my appetite for fruitful activity and for a high quality of life. Whatever time was left, whether it was a year or a decade, would be more than just a duration. I would continue to help the clots and clusters of withered and wretched in Asia to the utmost of my ability. The words of Camus rang through, "In the midst of winter I suddenly found that there was in me an invincible summer."

Maybe I could now be tender in a better way. I was a member of the fellowship of those who know the mark of pain. The philosophical concept of Dr. Schweitzer that he used to talk to me about years ago was now a more vivid thing—I bore that mark.

The days went on and on. The hospital had a monotony to it, though there was some turmoil in my hospital room. MEDICO had to set up an independent office. We had formerly been a division of the International Rescue Committee. Now we were an independent organization. My return and the ensuing public interest in and contributions to MEDICO made the time right. On September first we became MEDICO, Inc.

Now we had to get offices, typewriters, stationery, employees and a thousand other things. Mr. Zeckendorf gave us a suite of rooms in the Graybar Building at a dollar a year, though I told him I was willing to pay two bucks. The Metropolitan Life Insurance Company gave us much office furniture. Our typewriters were given to us. The Soundscriber Company donated their wonderful battery-run dictating machines to us. All around the country once again people were helping us to help others help themselves. MEDICO's administrative overhead would therefore be extremely low.

The days were busy with dressing changes, inoculations, examinations and all the things that make hospital life far from restful. One night I was all scrunched up in bed, the dressings on my legs tight and sore, my ankle swollen, my back aching from having to sit in bed so long, and my chest a mass of dressings from the belly up over the shoulders. The bed was bent in a "V" and I was lying over on one side, far, far from comfortable. Using an instrument panel I was able to push one button and turn on the television set. I got the John Daly newscast. He flashed on the screen a picture of me taken many months before and said "Dr. Dooley is resting comfortably tonight in Memorial Hospital." I quickly pushed the button off and wished the announcer could see how "comfortably" I was resting.

But when the night came and the peaceful silence once again flooded my room, my mind returned to my high valley. I could close my eyes and conjure up the village placidly floating before me like a Chinese landscape wrapped in a fine blue mist. I sometimes felt that familiar, cloudy out-of-touchness, that pleasant disembodiment from my own self. The physical tiredness after surgery melted away into liquid. I could see once again the mountains of my beloved northern Laos, its gulfs and gorges, the hosts of billowing clouds that roll off the slopes of the high rain forest. I could see the green lush valleys, and see huddled in their thatched huts, the sick of Laos. The valleys become gray green in the evening sun. The mountains disappear in the sunset glare—and it seems as though the sun itself thunders drily, before the rains begin.

I could see, from my cool quiet bed in America, the sickness of the valleys where I knew my boys were working now in the depths of the rains. I could see the whole side of the mountain heave and slither. The monsoon landscape. The waterlogged sodden land of Laos buried beneath the rains of heaven.

Convalescence from any kind of surgery can be an exhilarating phenomenon, lifting out of depression into a state of health. Often I would think of the boys, and one day a letter came through from them. It was dated Muong Sing, August 26, and I thought to myself that a plane must have come into the valley very soon after I left in order to get it to me in the second week of September. It was the first letter from the boys since I had left North Laos. I found out that they had known all this time that I had cancer. Dwight, when returning from Cambodia August 6th, had seen Bob Burns and Hank Miller in Vientiane. They had been notified by Dr. Van Valin after the specimen Van took to Bangkok was diagnosed by microscopy. The three of them decided that it would best *not* to tell me I had cancer. Knowing I was going home in October anyway, they thought (correctly so) that I would probably refuse to rush right home upon receipt of Dr. Comanduras' cable. So they kept it a secret from me. Dwight's letter explained their feelings:

Dear Sir:

Just a personal note to ask you to forgive us for having to practice a deception on you. I am sure you know that it had to be done that way or we would not have done it. At the time we felt right about it and if we had it to do over again, we would do it just the same. However, it was hard, very hard.

I knew it was doubly hard on them because they not only had to make the decision to get me out, but they had to make their decision as to whether they would stay on alone or not. They made their decision. They are fine men! The letter went on to say,

What I want to say is this: We are more proud than you will ever realize at being members of the first MEDICO team out in the field. As a result of this pride we intend to fill your shoes to the best of our ability until you come back here, as you certainly will. Earl and I want you to concentrate on getting well, and not upon worrying about your hospital. We promise you that you will never have to worry about any action of ours bringing anything but credit to you and to MEDICO. We realize that there are unbridgeable chasms that separate us. We realize that because of our relationship within the team we can never really be intimate friends. But we want you to know that we admire you greatly. We do or else we would all be back in the United States.

You know full well that we don't agree with you from time to time, but we hope you realize that if we didn't have the courage to disagree with you, we would not be men. And if we were not men, we would be of little use to you here in Laos.

It was signed with a Spanish expression that Dwight used so often, "*Anda con Dios.*"

I missed them very much. It is easier to part with the dead than the living. How profound my depth of admiration was for these boys. I knew they were doing well, and I heard later that they really didn't need me at all. I had worked myself out of a job.

My immediate plans were not muddled. I knew what I had to do. I had with me in the hospital the very beautiful letter that I had received from Dr. Charles Mayo informing me that I was to receive the Mutual of Omaha's Criss Award. I had received this letter in Laos in June, and it said,

Dr. Dooley, we are honoring you because of your outstanding contributions to the medically underprivileged peoples of the world. You have been an outstanding example of a free man helping other free men on a person-to-person basis. With this in mind, the Board of Judges has selected you as recipient of the 1959 Mutual of Omaha, Criss Award.

The letter had gone on to say that the Award would be given in Omaha on the 10th of November, and that they would pay for my ticket. Of course, I came home earlier for cancer and Mutual of Omaha paid for the ticket anyway.

Now I knew what I would do. I would spend the next couple of weeks in New York after discharge from the hospital. And then, as soon as possible, I would go out to Hawaii for my convalescence. In Hawaii I intended to give some speeches, make some money, and also write this book. I would return to America and go on a lecture tour. On November 10th I would go to Omaha to receive the Award, give a few more weeks of lectures, and then in December return to my high valley. I intended to be "home" in Laos for Christmas. I was.

When Dr. McNeer came in I told him of my plans and he gasped, "Well, if all dressings are finished and if the graft does not slough off, and if all goes well, I suppose there is really no reason that you can't." He knew as well as I that the internal "get up and fight" is half the battle against cancer. I had no intention to lie in a hospital bed and wither away. There was too much to do in this world. There is a line from a poem that my father gave to me long ago. It hung in my room as a child and said, " I must fill each minute full of sixty seconds' worth of distance run." On the night of the eighth day after my operation, I was discharged. They let me out at this time because I was very anxious to go to the United Nations on Labor Day.

The tiny Kingdom of Laos, to which I had devoted so much time and love, had brought its newest malady to the highest court on earth, the United Nations. The war was continuing in the provinces, the areas all around Earl and Dwight were aflame.

The government of Laos had sent a letter to the United Nations requesting that they investigate the situation in Laos, and bring to the attention of the whole world the fact that she was being invaded by outside forces.

The Secretary General, Dag Hammarskjold, called for an emergency meeting of the United Nations Security Council on Labor Day, an unprecedented thing. It made all of America wonder whether Laos would become another Korea. Would the land of Laos become the battleground where once again the blood of the young men of the world would be spilled? The Secretary General was in South America, but returned as speedily as possible to New York in time to preside at the special session of the Security Council on September 7, 1959–Labor Day. Dag Hammarskjold pointed out that the Lao plea was for the dispatch, as speedily as possible, of an emergency force to "halt aggression and to prevent its spreading." He pointed out that this was the first time in history that a specific request for action had been addressed to a main United Nations organ. Mr. Hammarskjold went on to indicate that the request of the Lao Government of the 4th of September confronted the United Nations with problems entirely different from any they had been confronted with so far. Would the UN respond immediately and precisely to the request of Laos, and dispatch an emergency force? Would it send a sub-committee, or an observer? Or would the UN merely get involved in a war of words, and help never emerge from the air-conditioned splendor of the conference halls on the East River?

I was able to secure a seat in the press section (I told them I represented the Bamboo Press of Muong Sing). Swathed in bandages from knee to nipple (I have only one left), I hobbled into the UN building on that fateful day. There were thousands of people standing outdoors waiting to get in. The whole world was focused upon the UN. Henry Cabot Lodge of the United States said that this plea from Laos was an appeal "which put us to the test." He went on to say that the appeal of a small state member such as Laos, which told of threats to its integrity by forces from the outside, could not be ignored. The United States had no doubt that aggression was being committed. The United States believed that Laos was a victim of this aggression and Mr. Lodge proposed a step to prevent spreading of the fires of war. In fact he went on to point out that there should be an emergency meeting that night, if necessary. He said that if the Security Council "presented to the world a spectacle of haggling and hair-splitting," the effectiveness of the UN would be greatly diminished.

The Security Council is a magnificent room. Seated before me were some of the great men in the world, representatives of England, France, Japan, Canada, Argentina, Tunisia, and many other countries. Here also was the Russian representative. Would he be able to block the adoption of the resolution?

Many hours were spent that afternoon while the Russian representative pointed out reasons why the resolution, in fact the whole Laos situation, could not legally be put on the agenda. However, by fine footwork and verbal skill, Mr. Lodge won out and indeed the question was put on the agenda.

I sat up in the balcony and looked at these people, in the glory of this magnificent building. I looked at the heavy drapes, the fine paintings, the thick rugs. But these are not the real marks of the greatness of the United Nations.

The whole magnificence of the United Nations is based upon a concept of the importance of the individual. Chai, Si, Ngoan, and my Kha Kho tribesmen were just as important as these delegates. This made me realize how wonderful it is to be a member of the community of free nations. How wonderful it is to see the free men of the world taking on themselves the responsibility of those in the world who are not free, who are threatened. The nation of Laos is small, obscure, and primitive. We all knew that Laos was being attacked by forces from without, but it is a hard thing to prove this against clever enemies. It is a hard thing to prove from just what area come the soldiers who pour down the high mountain valleys of North Laos. It is hard to "prove" anything in such a primitive land as this.

Had I seen in the future, I would have realized that before the end of November the whole Laos crisis would have quieted down, and the threat of war held off by firm action. America did a good job. Laos did a better one. The UN showed herself capable of answering a challenge.

The American Government stood by its promises to help safeguard the integrity of Laos. In September the small units that had been crossing the borders in Sam Neua and Phong Saly began to pull back. Everyone thought the town of Sam Neua would fall, yet in the next few days it was obvious that the Pathet Lao forces had received a pull-back order. We had shown Laos that we did indeed intend to back her. As one newspaper put it that very night: "Fingers crossed, in short, we can say that the Free World has had a significant success. Laos is free, and will probably maintain her freedom. America has stood by a threatened nation. We have shown ourselves to be the great nation of love and care for our brothers we profess that we are."

I knew that I would have to go on a lecture tour and once again try to raise money and men and medicines. MEDICO, Inc. with hospitals and programs now in nine nations should grow and grow. We need the awareness and the dollar support of all men. I knew that I would return to Laos, and would indeed be home for Christmas. But first I still had three months in the States. My mountain was not burned. Yes, but new life was planted in my heart. My night was now day. I must strive once again to help achieve that dream of Anne Frank's, "Things will change, and men become good again, and these pitiless days will come to an end, and the world will know once again order, trust, and peace."

I left the UN just as the sun was setting, hailed a cab and asked to be taken to my hotel. The driver adjusted the mirror, looked back at me and said, "You been at the UN, aintcha, Mac?" I said yes. He said, "You've seen a lot of Communism, aintcha?" I said yes. He adjusted the mirror and looked at me again, studying my face and the way I was hunched over in the back seat, just as he had watched the stiffness with which I had climbed into his taxi. Evidently he recognized me. As we pulled up to the hotel the fare was eighty cents and I gave the driver a dollar. He looked at me, thrust the dollar bill back in my hand and said, "Oh never mind, Dr. Dooley, I'll pay your fare. You keep that buck and get back as soon as possible to your kingdom of Laos." I smiled and felt warm and good inside and turned to my fellow-American and said, "O.K., Mac. Shall do."